THE STA
SCHIZOPHRENIA

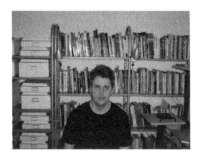

BY Mark Ellerby

"One million people commit suicide every year."
The World Health Organization

Published by:
Chipmunkapublishing
PO Box 6872
Brentwood
Essex
CM13 1ZT
United Kingdom

http://www.chipmunkapublishing.com

Proof-read by Ben Vickers

INTRODUCTION

Schizophrenia – A personal experience.

At age 21, life could not be better. I had just graduated from University with a first class degree, had been accepted to study for a doctorate with funding (perhaps the academic equivalent of being selected for the Olympic team) and had a research supervisor who was a member of the House of Lords. What could go wrong?

Nothing, or so it seemed. Then it happened: Schizophrenia. It was not a sudden shock, more of a gradual onset, although nothing had prepared me for it. Nobody takes you aside at school and says, "Look you might get a mental illness!" There was no information available to allow a self-diagnosis. I had heard of Schizophrenia, but thought it was a split or dual personality. It was all the more frightening back then as I didn't know how to help myself.

For the first few years, I stayed at university in Southampton; the opposite end of the country and away from home and family. I managed to keep my head above water on my course, as the symptoms were not so bad at the start. I kept hearing people talking about my actions, behaviour and thoughts. Eventually I spent more time thinking about this than my work and had to give it up and go home – just in time.

My psychiatrist described my symptoms as particularly severe so they are probably worth recounting. I kept hearing the neighbours banging on the walls trying to play on my nerves (or so I thought). My response was to run not just out of the house, but to get as far away as possible. That meant getting away from everybody. I wandered round the countryside at night trying to avoid towns and villages from which direction I could still hear the banging noise. I had paranoia and auditory hallucinations all mixed together.

This however was not the end of the matter. I had other kinds of delusions. I thought I was responsible for all kinds of problems such as wars, crime and disease. The worst such symptom was that I had memories of being the reason why everything from TV programmes to the architecture of buildings had the form and appearances they did. It was like wandering around in my own subconscious. I tried 'ump-teen' times to commit suicide but was sectioned and taken to hospital.

I was in there for more than a year while 'They'; the doctors, tried to find the right drug. The illness never was a continual thing – I had good periods and bad. I was then put on Risperidone and some of the delusional symptoms seemed to improve. I still had other problems, most notably strange thoughts and periodic head pains but I think the doctors must have thought that by then I had gone through the system and come out the other side!

I was left to live independently. That proved very difficult. The stigma of mental illness made me a virtual recluse. You cannot go down the pub and face the inevitable question; "what do you do?" and reply you are schizophrenic. On my own, the presence of the voices seemed to be magnified and there was little to help the depression this created. The answer was to live in sheltered accommodation, and as with my stay in hospital, this improved things further.

What I have learned about having such an illness is that one of the best things that can be done is to simply talk to the patient. I guess this can act as a distraction and prevent you from dwelling on your problems. Living together in sheltered housing aims to provide such a context. Some kind of activity is also necessary but this can be a double-edged sword; work can be stressful but then doing nothing can be the same so it is often necessary to balance the two. Variety, in terms of people and activity, is also necessary.

The biggest help in my case seems, at present, to be the drug Clozapine. My mental health has greatly improved since the very first time it was prescribed to me. That was two years ago! I still have some symptoms and side effects but I am now a thousand times better. I have started to research and write again, this time about mental health. To date I have had a lot of publishing success. I guess the lesson here is that every cloud has a 'silver lining', so keep hoping.

Mark Ellerby, 2005.

A Schizophrenic life.

I sometimes reflect on the sad side of schizophrenia.

Schizophrenia usually begins in the early twenties. This is often not at an age when you have had a chance to get married and have children. Do I regret not being married? Actually, I like being single. Personally too, the worry of having a family and kids (who may be taken off you by social services) is avoided.

Yet being young free and single could be seen as the best time in ones life, although as Robbie Williams sings "Youth is wasted on the young. Before you know it, it has come and gone too soon". Thus some people think life begins at 40. I will tell you what I think when I get there!

Some people too say your school days are the best days of your life. A time when you do not have any real worries or responsibilities. In my case, I spent so much time doing homework at school I cannot really say it was worth it, as it did not come to fruition career wise. No body warns you that you might get a mental illness.

Being married or in a relationship is itself a responsibility. I have had a schizophrenic girl friend but when she was ill it did not drag me down with her. Thus, I think it is possible to be married and very ill. This is very encouraging

Personal Experiences - A case study.

It is often said that schizophrenia cannot be understood unless you have had it yourself. I would not go so far as to say it is unimaginable, but the problem of communicating the experience requires an in depth look at a particular case. I believe it is possible to communicate it a little more than this first sentence indicates.

Metaphor is often the starting point of such description. Schizophrenia is a journey to hell and back. It is a nightmare, the end of the world or walking alone through the shadow of the valley of death. This I think is the common understanding; that it is an extremely frightening experience. The problem is how to explain why.

It is what could be described as a kind mystery. How could such being or existence be known? It is what Foucault defined as 'the other.' Something which can only be known if you.have had it yourself. We can perhaps relate to the fear aspect most easily.

I think there is too much concentration on the fear aspect because it is so visible. Furthermore, we all have experienced anxiety and fear to some extent, but I wonder if many people really do know about this sort of fear?

I do not experience the same level of fear all the time. This fear is something that can paralyse you.

Sometimes I cannot get out of bed, sometimes I cannot get out of my room and sometimes I cannot get out of the building.

When fear is connected to paranoia, i.e. the thought, particularly in public places, that everyone is watching you. This feels a little like stage fright. You are under the spotlight and are the focus of attention. There is a fascination with such fear - why is it that I am the centre of attention? It is not altogether a bad feeling.

Fear can be addictive too. Rather like bungee jumping; it is exciting even to the point that I believe you can get addicted to the schizophrenic experience, providing it is not all the time.

Another analogy I find rather interesting is that it is a little like being a soldier in the Vietnam War. You are never sure when someone is going to jump out at you. This is not because I was afraid someone was going to shoot at me, but simply that there are long intervals where nothing happened. These were followed by short terrifying periods of vivid delusions, during which I thought I was going to be killed.

The next thought in the psychiatrist's mind (it seems to me) is 'what is causing this fear?' In my case, I thought that I was going to die when I was 30. At that deadline, I would be held responsible for all the woes of the world, that it was all my fault and I would be punished. This definitely made me 'afraid', but I was also afraid of committing suicide. In the end, I ended up trying to avoid thinking about it all and hoping it would go away. This took some time and I kept just trying to muddle through.

How I actually managed this, I will never know. It was certainly not because I was brave or managed to find a way to cope which I could pass on to other people. I simply existed in this state of being as the days endlessly came and went.

After noting the reasons for the fear, medication is prescribed and you are put in hospital notionally for your own protection. I did not feel any safer in hospital than at home. The surroundings were less familiar with new people and places and I ended up thinking at one point that they were all just there to terrorise me further. I still associate the buildings and people with my paranoia and can still feel very uncomfortable near them. However, to me the interesting thing about my experience was not fear, but it's cause.

Psychiatrists sometimes think of delusions in a causal and negative way. They are merely the result of a chemical imbalance. It is forbidden to collude with the patient in respect of these delusions. To the patient the causes and consequences are not foremost in his or her mind, rather it is their thoughts and it their impact on their lives. This can be positive or negative, but it is all the same to the psychiatrist.

I have found it useful to balance the negative and the positive in order to measure up the situation I found myself. This is only natural, if think you are in trouble or responsible for atrocities etc. It was like balancing the scales of justice. It was also a response to try to justify it all, but the more I thought about it the more complex it all became. In the end, I gave up the attempt.

I also moved in and out of the delusional phases, but this did not help me recognise their unreality. I can only compare the lucid and vivid clarity of these thoughts to a religious revelation. It was like a vision appearing in my minds eye. It struck me like a 'bolt of lightening', but started panicking me instead of going into shock. Each time it happened, it was real even in spite of the intervening periods.

I could not talk about it because I did not know what to say. This was initially because I was 'dumb struck', but how do you describe that sort of thing? It opens up a whole new world. It starts you on a journey characterised by day-to-day survival and in my case; not knowing what is going to happen to you next. It can change your identity, your beliefs and attachments. The first feeling I think you get with all this is the newness of everything and that everything is changing.

In this world, you have to adjust to the new circumstances. You will have new beliefs and attitudes to weigh up, new facts about yourself and new opinions on how others perceive you. Furthermore, you need to get over the strangeness of it all. You can remember before the meta-morphosis however, it is 'the change' you focus on. Any change (such as moving house) is stressful, but changing your whole world is a veritable "sea change" and belongs to a different category altogether. Delusions can be very stressful and may cause a nervous breakdown and/or depression without fear.

There was one peculiarity in my case that I am able to describe in more detail. I have not encountered elsewhere and is worth a mention because of its severity. I used to think I was in terrible pain. This was not a delusion but a sensory hallucination - I could actually feel it. The pain was even present whilst I was hearing voices etc. I ended up thinking the two were connected. This seemed to me to give my symptoms an added reality. I often wondered if it was a side effect but the doctors said otherwise.

I had a hard time convincing everyone that my head pain was real. Often, I would get a headache at the same time as a frightening thought. How could they be related? Thoughts are mental, pain is physical. The only way to deal with it and the concurrent thoughts was to take a sleeping tablet and usually by the morning, the pain and the thoughts were gone.

This happened quite frequently, each time was a nightmare, but I found myself anticipating the next episode during the time I had in between. This often kept my mood low. I kept wondering how this could happen? I could not find a sensible answer. I even thought that god was trying to punish me, this may have suggested to the doctors that the whole thing was even more delusional!

Every time this happened, I had to go to sleep which disrupted my personal and social relationships.
I ended up being housebound. I was afraid to go out because you cannot sit on a bus and start reeling around on the floor in pain. People would wonder what was going on. In the end, I thought I could say that I had a migraine and so began to venture outside.

At my worst point, I started screaming and had to call out my consultant (not the on-call psychiatrist but the top doctor) in the middle of the night to assess me. My vocal chords were hoarse, I couldn't lie still because of the imagined pain and I was thinking that I had lost control of my mind.

Eventually it went away. To this day, I still wonder 'how?' and 'why?' It is amazing how quickly you can forget even an experience like this. Going into hospital made the symptoms worse at first and I ended up being in there for six months. Eventually things improved and learned to rely on the nurses for help.

All this means is that I have been in and out of hospital with differing symptoms. I was even in the lock-up ward a few times. This is the intensive therapy unit and not a ward for violent patients. My experience of this was that it felt quite cosy! To this extent, it was therapeutic. However, the small spatial confines did feel very restrictive and I genuinely felt 'locked up.' When I was released, I could almost smell a sense of freedom and liberation.

My 'psychiatric history' is thus a mixed picture. I have had different symptoms at different times. First voices, then delusions, after that I had these plus strange occipital pain and then periodic repetitions of these symptoms in different combinations. Also at one point, I felt I was doing so well I had all but recovered only for the same symptoms to come back. Now I feel as though they are unlikely to ever go away completely, so my emphasis now is discovering how to live with my delusions and paranoia.

Trying to get off a section.

Any appeal against a section is taken very seriously since your basic human rights and liberties are taken very seriously. It involves getting an independent psychiatrist to interview you. You get your own Lawyer.
However, the onus is on the patient to try and prove they are capable of judging their own well being in order to overturn the section. The burden of proof does not lie with the psychiatrist.

The first thing that struck me was the number of people involved. Having been ill, I did not like the feeling of being under the spotlight. I definitely had stage fright. The panel is composed of a chairman (who is a lawyer), another psychiatrist and a lay person being trained in mental health matters.

The whole thing felt like sitting your 'A Levels'. The interview I had was quite arduous. It lasted three hours. It was very detailed with lots of questions. I had to formulate everything I wanted to say at the end of the interview and then wait for the result. My lawyer helped with the former and was just as nervous as I was about the latter!

I must have looked pretty tired at the end of the three hours which I think went against me. It was however, very unusual (it was pointed out to me) for the assessment to take that long. I think I may have been treated a little unfairly in this respect.

You were not allowed to speak whilst the commission questioned the different professionals. They went right back through my psychiatric history and the circumstances of the section. My social worker, psychiatrist, and my link worker nurse all had to submit detailed reports which were then picked over with a fine tooth comb. I had to remember all the points made in this process to argue my case against each one. This is extremely difficult when your ill and you definitely need a good lawyer (mine was excellent).

My main argument was that I would stay in hospital voluntarily but during my psychotic episodes, I would want to go home. This was buttressed by the fact that I had previously been in hospital for over a year, during which time I was mostly a voluntary patient. This was duly noted.

I think the panel psychiatrist felt I had some insight because I knew about the stigma of mental health and noted this down when I said it. At one of my sections my lawyer felt the lay person was also convinced that I was O.K. to leave hospital since he rudely asked me, "what were your plans for the future?" (I replied that I just wanted to go back to university to finish my PhD).

In my case, the independent psychiatrist actually supported my appeal even though I was very ill. However, I was told that although I interacted or 'presented' myself (as they put it) normally, my symptoms could still deteriorate very quickly and I could quickly become very ill. The nurse at the inquest even said that a section was not needed on a day-to-day basis, but only at the periodic moments when such an episode occurred. Hence, in the end despite having medical opinion on my side, I still failed to get off the section.

At these times I occasionally tried to escape from hospital although this was only to run back home or to go to my parent's house. Once I was brought back, I was still allowed out of the hospital grounds on leave the following day. The commission looked at this seeming paradox very closely and asked many questions about it. What they made of it, I can only guess.

If you have a history of 'non-compliance' with medication, then this will go against you. This was supposed to be the case with me and my parents supported the view that I was getting ill only during the moments in which I forgot to take them. I was never really sure if simply missing the occasional dose could trigger this and, to be honest, I still question it sometimes.

My main criticism of the process is that in appealing to get off a section takes a long time to arrange - ten weeks. After that, you can appeal to the mental health commission to review it after six months. I believe this is far too long and should be (at most) three months and then a further appeal at six months. On the whole, looking back I think that they were correct in my case but then that's looking back. At the time, it felt like confinement.

A day in the life of a Schizophrenic.

The first notable thing is getting up in the morning, although sometimes you wake up in the afternoon. My first thought often is how well you sleep as a result of the sedation. Do I feel refreshed? Not often because from the moment you are awake, `it` immediately hits you. You are thinking that you are the cause of war, famine and disease. From the moment you are awake you can be paralysed with fear.

This paralysis can last for up to a few hours. Then you begin to move. Once this is possible you might be able to take some diazepam (nerve tablets). This calms your body down, but your mind is still focused on the delusions, so much so that you do not even realise how depressing living like this actually is.

Having got this far, the next step is to decide whether to open the curtains or not. This is difficult in case people are watching you. Living in the dark for a week or two inside a house without social contact is like a spell in solitary confinement in prison and adds stress to the list of daily problems. Nevertheless, it is possible to cope with this, as I shall now explain.

The first thing to do is to try to distract yourself if you are able to calm down enough. I have a vast library of compact disks, DVD films and computer games. These are a kind of psychological fortification against intrusive thoughts and voices since they can help you whilst you are at home and indoors.

Obviously living this way creates other problems. If you go into hibernation for a week, how do you get your shopping in? The internet comes in very useful here as you can order it from a supermarket online. Failing that, your local pizza outlet comes in very useful due to it being at the end of a phone line. You still have to sound normal on the phone, which is not at all easy.

Another daily problem is remembering your medication. This might seem a strange subject to write about as if you stop taking it you become ill. Nurses can give you medication but only when it is prescribed by a doctor. It is easier to get a depot injection that lasts for a month, however this is undesirable because it has more side effects.

It is also easy to abuse the medication. By this, I do not mean getting addicted to it. Rather the sedatives in the anti-psychotic drugs seem about ten times more powerful than sleeping tablets. The temptation is there to use this even instead of the Vallium so that you can simply sleep through the worst of it.

At other times when the symptoms are less severe, it is possible to venture outside. This is OK if I am going somewhere where everybody knows me and understands my problems. However, getting on a bus whilst appearing very nervous (or at worst getting a panic attack) is a major obstacle. It is much easier to get a taxi, sometimes I feel I have no choice but to do this.

Thankfully, these symptoms are not present all the time so it is up to the individual to make the most of the good times. The trouble here is that you learn to associate going out with being ill therefore you end up with a psychological barrier that interferes with such an attempt. In my case this has to be repeatedly overcome before I get back to 'normal.'

Having got out of the building you need to decide where to go. This could be a variety of places. Somewhere without too many people around (say a walk through some remote pathway) seems the obvious choice but is seldom chosen. This is because social contact is needed most. This therefore means getting to my local mental health day centre.

If my family is present, this could also mean a trip to my local shopping mall for some retail therapy. I never get sick of this and come back on a high. However, the high cannot last forever when waiting round the corner (so to speak) is the next bout of delusional fear.

Life then is strangely full of ups and downs and is not at all negative. The point is to try to brave these symptoms step by step, I have now even got off the diazepam (which is also very addictive). It is still early days, but I will let you know how it all pans out.

The first beginnings of Schizophrenia - 1994.

The initial onset of schizophrenia in my case was very gradual. I started hearing voices. They were quiet. I only heard them every now and again. At first, it was possible to ignore them and I managed to hold down a couple of jobs. However, the longer it went on and without an increase in frequency, they came to dominate all my thinking. This was because it was coupled with a rather vague feeling that I was losing touch with reality at the same time. I associated the voices with my suspicions about the world having a strange 'dream like' quality. At no point in the process did I associate what was happening with schizophrenia.

I thought that people could read my mind and that I had recently discovered this faculty, so I went to ask my parents about it. They said straight off; "I want you to tell a doctor exactly what you are telling me." So I did. The doctor's response was; "I think the idea that people can discern thoughts is an incredible suggestion." This was closely followed by; "you seem to have schizophrenia." I was so ignorant of the condition I replied; "can you die from it?" The doctor laughed at this suggestion.

However, the question was very serious. I looked up the word "schizophrenia" to find it meant, "Split mind." This gave me the impression that the two halves of the brain might divide, severing any interconnection and killing the patient in the process! Looking back, I do not think doctors should be allowed to make a diagnosis with a label like that due to it having too many social connotations.

Sometime later, the voices became more intrusive and the strange unreality of the world turned into terrifying delusions. This whole process took about five years. I would say looking back, the voices were about as frightening as the delusions. I had to go to the doctor for a sick note for depression (I had heard about that!). Without work, I became more and more isolated from society and cut off from life.

In the end I could not survive by myself and tried to move back in with my parents. I lived just round the corner but could not stand the slum I was living in. Spurred on by this and the voices, I used to go for long walks that lasted all night! When my parents eventually found out they called the fell rescue and I ended up in the national newspapers.

Thus, it all got too difficult to bear so I was sectioned and taken to hospital. I did not really think I was 'ill' and tried to resist. The police were called and eventually I saw sense. I went peacefully, but only after a section was imposed on me. I was taken away in an ambulance and gave in to all the pressure because I was so mentally tired by the whole experience.

Hospital really worked for me and I was eventually

discharged. Now I think if I ever have to go back again I would go voluntarily.

First contacts with a psychiatrist.

There may be some resistance on the part of the patient to being interviewed. Why should I tell you about my problems? It is necessary to sell the concept of being mentally ill.

Hospital design is part of the process. In the one I attend, there is coffee available, music playing and art on the walls. The informality of the staff is also important. Plus attention to how psychiatrists and nurses dress casually? First impressions, or are we too ill to notice? What more can be done to get the message across? Is it all in vain?

The answer here is no. I think people who constantly care for emotionally distressed people demonstrate an ethos of care that manifests itself in the being and behaviour of nurses and doctors. This in my hospital is so visible; the above considerations seem to fade into the background.

If the patient closes themselves off to the staff then a relationship of trust and confidence will be harder to establish. You might, if you are not aware of these influences (e.g. because you are so caught up by the illness), feel like you are just a part of the system rather than an individual in the eyes of the staff. This is not true.

If I were more aware of the buildings, I would have wondered a little about the notorious carcarel history of psychiatry. Although I am doubtful, newer buildings would help in this respect.

One important point is that they should know what they are doing when they label someone with 'schizophrenia.' Having a social worker on hand to explain about the media stigma and the connotations the word has, the negative language involved and how its all just ignorance in that respect. This is better than just saying it is a chemical imbalance, which may be enlightened only if we are properly educated in this respect. My parents felt there was a general lack of information about the subject.

I believe that when sectioned, you should have a lawyer on hand to supervise the process from the start. This might just help reassure the patient that their rights are not being infringed, although I am not altogether sure about this. However, if the police are involved in a crime you get one so why not for mental health?

I think hospital can be a good thing in respect of educating relatives and sufferers because you are in a medical institution and thus the idea that you have an illness is inescapable. Alternatively, home visits could introduce the subject in less confusing surroundings. By this, I mean the hospital buildings bring a rather vague and confused picture of 'mental health' as opposed to 'physical health' to mind but do not always help by doing this. At the limit I think both approaches have their merits but a home visit then a day unit appointment might be the best introduction to the system.

We educate teenagers about war in schools so why not schizophrenia? It is just about as frightening. In the end some kind of public programme is needed to underpin initial psychiatric contact.

When I was first labelled with 'schizophrenia' I had a subconscious fear of it and although I was dimly aware of its existence, my immediate reaction was to ask "what is that?" I had heard of it but it was not in the forefront of my mind that it was an illness at all. After a couple of weeks the medical aspect dawned on me. I decided to do some research in the library. This was the worst thing to do; a little knowledge is dangerous. I found it literally meant split mind, what could that possibly mean?

A day unit is a much better place to learn about mental illness than a G.P.'s Surgery. There are notice boards everywhere advertising 'Mind', web sites, self help groups and information on therapies etc.

Ultimately, I don't think the word 'schizophrenia' should now be used at all. It may be better to simply describe it as 'paranoia' and of hearing voices as 'hallucinating'. These terms are not ideal but they are far more innocuous than the words 'schizophrenia' or 'psychosis'. By way of contrast,

I think 'depression' is an excellent term and far clearer than 'mood disorder'.

Perhaps some people who cope with particularly severe schizophrenia should even be awarded the Victoria Cross? This is the best public defence against the stigma. What the future holds in the age of science and robotics, more than bravery; is intelligence? Mental health and the associated stigma are vital here. However, the illness destroys what could be a fertile mind, the best surety for the progress of societies.

Symptoms of Schizophrenia.

Some of the more severe symptoms of schizophrenia, for instance thinking the neighbours are persecuting them, sometimes involve drawing the curtains to stop the neighbours spying or perhaps crawling underneath windows to move around, go to the toilet etc. This is a very graphic example of what schizophrenia can be like, however there are many other symptoms. Some of the most common are described below.

One is the belief that people are talking about one self. Quite often we might get the idea someone is calling you and so say "I could have sworn I heard … etc." after realising the mistake. This is all the more beguiling, when the actual as opposed to the imagined voices manifest themselves in the same way. What I think can sometimes give lie to this is the frequency of such instances; some schizophrenics hear voices eighty per cent of the day.

When, you are paranoid, life goes on around you seemingly as normal. It is a paradox that is sometimes difficult to explain. However, it is perhaps best described by, the admittedly rather vague notion, that it has an air of unreality about it. This takes the form of a rather vague subjective feeling. None the less, it is probably the most accurate account of all that goes on in the mind of the schizophrenic.

You can also remember a time before the illness began, when you did not think like this. Some sort of reason or cause however, can sometimes explain this seeming paradox. The longer such an illness goes on however, the harder it is to remember what life was like 'back then.' Despite this, what does seem to stick in the memory is the abrupt change that begins at the start of the illness, although the onset can sometimes be very gradual.

Not all such symptoms are a direct result of psychoses however. If someone smiles it could be thought that they are laughing at one's self. Such beliefs can thus be challenged by other equally plausible explanations in order to gain some 'insight'. The difficulty is that we must know which are straight forwardly psychotic and which are mistaken interpretations, even though they may seem to fit the facts. Sometimes, things can seem real until we question them.

The experience of schizophrenia generally seems fantastical to 'sane' people, to the point that delusional beliefs are 'comical' because they defy common sense. A little thought however, can reveal how insipid such beliefs really are. Take for example the schizophrenic's very common idea that people are persecuting you. In the schizophrenic mind, the persecution of Jews (which occurred in a country so very close, so civilised and so very culturally similar to Britain as

Germany) could be taken as evidence. There are many other examples in the west, such as the brutal purges by Stalin in Russia, not to mention the treatment of British P.O.W.'s by the Japanese. Indeed it was not the British who invented concentration camps?

Another related and typical schizophrenic belief is the thought that someone is trying to kill you. Again, this is something that is not impossible however strange it may seem to other people. Indeed, any such allegation is certainly taken very seriously by the police if it is reported to them. But here again, look at the frequency of murder mysteries and police dramas in the media compared to actual such acts in society. This again magnifies any thought of conspiracy, plotting, ill will or harmful intentions etc.

Another common schizophrenic symptom is the thought that people are talking about them on the television or radio. This often seems to confuse people who have no experience of the illness. How can the script of a soap opera or the lyrics to a song be directed at someone in particular, when it is not actually what the words say or the person is unnamed or identified? The answer simply, is that we can relate to the lyrics in songs and the characters in dramas. They either directly or indirectly become about oneself, despite the fact that they are also about everyone else as well.

Anyone who has had long-term experience of

schizophrenia has also experienced one or more of these symptoms with the confusion and perplexity this entails. As the psychiatrist in 'A Beautiful Mind' starring Russell Crowe pointed; "the nightmare of schizophrenia, is that we are unable to distinguish the real from the imagined".

Masquerade.

How the symptoms of schizophrenia can masquerade as one another and as other illnesses.

I have had two bouts of full blown or 'acute' schizophrenia and both times I have had to go to hospital because of it. What sticks in my mind most about these times, apart from being really ill, is that looking back I have often wondered what the precise symptoms were. This might seem peculiar because though schizophrenia is just about hearing voices and having paranoid delusions, it is (as we all know) different for everyone.

A lot depends on what the voices say. In my case, they said I was responsible for wars, crime and diseases. However, this was what I had been having delusions about before hearing the voices. Thus the two came to interact and reinforce each other. It may even have been that the voices were saying that they was all my fault. As a result I came to believe such things anyway without being 'delusional' at all.

Often if you hear voices whilst being delusional, this can suggest to the patient that instead of being real, the delusional ideas may simply be other symptoms of the illness. This can be reinforced by the fact that other patients you meet in hospital also believe similar things. However, hearing voices can be a very beguiling thing. They can be so persuasive, that they can more or less 'brain wash' you into believing impossible things (in the same way religious cults are often accused of).

Another problem is that, as we all know, depression can go hand in hand with Schizophrenia. At the worst times I felt I had depression, but did not respond to the anti-depressant treatments. I never had this particular problem all the time, which has left me wondering whether the depression actually was just another delusion, i.e. that feeling depressed was all just in my head!

This is important because if one illness can masquerade as another, it implies a different regime of medication. I feel it important therefore to recount the above tale. On the other hand I might be thinking about it all too much. As Freud said; "sometimes a cigar is just a cigar"!

Delusions.

Having delusions can involve a multiplicity of interlocking details that sometimes interact with the other schizophrenic symptoms such as hearing voices or paranoia. All this can make up a delusion as well as giving it an added and sometimes terrifying 'reality'. What follows is one account of such a complex and panoramic experience.

Although the experience I am to describe, encompasses a diverse subject matter and to some extent different delusional beliefs, it all conforms to one general theme or set of underlying notions. Everyone will recognise these beliefs as 'delusions of grandeur' or 'paranoid delusions'. This is not the end of the matter however, as everybody's experience of these phenomena is different, despite the central place of these epithets in medical diagnosis. Sometimes however, it is not just the form of the illness but the content that is important.

The delusional notion involved is a long story. It in fact encompasses an entire lifetime of memories often revealed as flashbacks of events and experiences, conversations and coincidences that date back to early childhood. The delusion was also expansive in a different sense. It involved the notional invention and development of just about everything; from computers to houses, from music to cars. What tied all of this together was one central fixed idea – that of my persecution.

The point of this preamble is not to re-describe what are generally fairly ordinary schizophrenic symptoms, but to note an example of what can make them so terrifying. The cultural and historical elements of the delusion above were intimately bound up with the idea that one group in society was persecuting another and that I was the cause. The causes lay in my own personal history and the cultural inventions and designs were the symbols of conflict. Ultimately, I was to be held responsible for this persecution, which therefore meant it would all be done back to me. It was not that the neighbours were out to get me, it was the whole world! Why then was this so particularly frightening?

The experience was a little like that of Winston Smith in George Orwell's '1984'. One morning, I seemed to find myself in a world that was strange and totally different, where people and media talked in 'newspeak', where the past was erased, forgotten or renamed whilst every tree and lamppost contained a hidden camera or microphone to spy on me. The all-pervasive paranoia which society generates, is very similar to the experience of schizophrenia in general, whilst its newness is similar to the experience I am describing in particular.

In such a world we cannot trust anything – language, people and or even ourselves. Orwell famously defined this latter aspect 'The thought police'. Was it possible someone could tell what I was thinking? What would be the consequence of being held responsible for this? What horrors awaited me because of my thoughts and actions? How is it possible to control one's own thoughts? Was there any way to escape such surveillance? Crucially being schizophrenic in such a society can be like Orwell's notion of 'big brother is watching you.'

Also in Orwell's world, big brother had an outwardly friendly and smiling face, as do all such regimes. Thus in Orwell's world, surveillance was secret. However in contrast, in the experience I am narrating there were often more open threats and signs of what I imagined was going to happen to me. However, they were to some extent 'veiled threats' so as to perhaps increase the paranoia. The notion that the government is also 'out to get you' also formed a central part of the delusion I am narrating.

There were differences however. Orwell's character Winston Smith did not hear voices. It might be that this symptom could lead the otherwise deluded patient to the conclusion that they have schizophrenia. Unfortunately however, this is not always the case. Sometimes the individual concerned may think that they are psychic or even that they are receiving messages from transmitters. In my case, the interpretation was that the government was broadcasting voices to me. Even this seemed to fit with the rest of the 'scenario' I was presented with.

That was not the end of the matter. I also had tactile (sensory) hallucinations, namely strange headaches. These appeared strange because they were mostly triggered by comments made by other people but also the imaginary voices. The voices would present me with all sorts of reasons and arguments about why I was responsible for persecuting other people and why I was therefore going to be persecuted myself in turn. These voices were particularly clever at interpreting the symbols of this persecution within the cultural products outlined above that I believed I had invented.

These often took the form of subtle hints of what was going to happen to me rather than outright statements openly declaring the fact. For example, if it was about suicide or death, it could be contained in the lyrics of a song or the sound of a piece of music etc. There seemed to be a million such examples that surrounded me everywhere, allowing no possibility of escape or rest. I even thought of emigrating and tried to walk into the North Pennines believing the remoteness of the area would allow me sanctuary. I even tried the sanctuary knocker on the door of Durham Cathedral to the same effect!

But even in such a seemingly hopeless situation there was hope. This went on and on, and probably would have continued *ad infinitum* had I not noted something curious about it all, namely that year in and year out, the expected persecutory punishment failed to materialise. I began to wonder why? Like Russell Crowe in 'A beautiful mind' there was a discrepancy despite the obvious reality of the delusions. This could be a potential consideration for others with such problems however convincing they may appear. It seems to give much cause for hope 'inspite of everything'.

Hearing Voices.

It is often difficult to encourage a person who hears voices to talk about them socially. This is partly a result of stigma, but voices can be so frightening you just have to keep silent about them - period. Hence this account.

What most people who know anything about mental health, will generally imagine about the symptom is the fact that the voices can be fiercely critical. This can cause depression and suicide. If the voices are criticising a person, a psychotherapist will probably intervene by emphasising your good points. Sometimes however, 'cognitive therapy' does not work as voices can talk about many other things. It might for instance be the voice of God, or the voice of the Devil. Sometimes, it is not possible to confront or persuade the voices to go away. Thus the reality is that the experience can be so varied, it is impossible to generalise. I will therefore have to concentrate mostly on my own experiences.

When I heard voices I also had other symptoms, for example being delusional about everything. In the solitude this created, the voices (although they were telling me things about the delusions) where nevertheless a *physical presence*. They were there with me when no one else was. Thus in a really weird way, they provided a distraction from my delusions to the point that I came to depend on hearing them. I would even go so far as to say they provided a kind of psychological security. I ended up wandering for miles around the countryside at night, yet time and physical distances seemed to fly by because I was so distracted by what I was hearing.

Another thought I often had was 'will the voices take control of me?' I used to hear voices telling me to burn my house down, so much so that I walked to a police station three miles away to have myself locked up. Naturally they did - not knowing what else to do! It is less than 1% of schizophrenics that are actually violent but I can see how it could happen. The medical staff at the time seemed to see this outcome as impossible, however it seemed pretty real to me. The real problem is that what you believe is in relation to what they say, you can be 'brain washed' if you prefer, and thus do as they instruct.

Medication can help with the nerves and depression you go through, but how far does that help with the experience? It is not something you ever really get used to. Unless you have experienced it yourself you will not know what it is like. The weirdest experience I have ever had was driving through the middle of nowhere and hearing voices despite nobody else being around for miles. Where do these voices come from? How can they affect me so far away from any other people?

Where does this voice come from? Another

question that preoccupied me. Paranoia thus sets in! The two main symptoms of schizophrenia, it seems to me, are definitely linked. Depression then sets in and your nerves go haywire. Hearing voices is often a package deal it seems to me - but that is not the worst of it.

The severity of the symptom seems to depend upon two things. Much depends, as I have outlined, upon the content of what you hear. The other is frequency. Some schizophrenics hear voices 80% of the day, day in day out, year in year out. The only graphic description I have ever come across that reflects the worst cases can be found in the lyrics of Slayer:

"voices inside my head pull me under, voices oppress like roaring thunder.
All this strife inside my brain, how much can I take of your pain."

I hope this provoke readers who have experienced such voices to record their experiences.

Depression

I have only had depression once and it lasted for only three months. Everything in my life at that point (aged 21) seemed to end concurrently. My parents' business went bankrupt, we were made homeless and I had a serious relationship that ended badly. Just when I thought things could not get any worse, shortly afterwards I got schizophrenia which could have been caused by stress.

During my period of depression I cried myself to sleep every night, something a man is not supposed to do. My nerves then gave up and I had a breakdown. The result was a kind of catastrophic shock to my system leaving me stunned by it all. I was scarcely aware of life and other people's lives going on around me - seemingly as normal.

Getting over that relationship took 10 years and I have had a few more relationships since, I now receive DLA and both my parents are remarried and comfortable. I would not say I am happy but I am more content now than a have been in a long time. So if it ever seems that there is no light at the end of the tunnel and you're painting the whole world black, hold on!

When I had depression, a Victorian idea that you are responsible alone for sorting your own life, made me keep quiet about my problems. I was thus unable to get help. Eventually due to this and other circumstances I moved back home. I was lucky that my parents knew more about this illness than me.

Looking back, I am absolutely convinced that depression is a medical condition just like a disease. I am still a little bit depressed even now and believe that tablets should be handed out like painkillers. Even if you are just sad because you have had an off day or the weather is dreary and so go shopping or out on the town, become irritable and argumentative with your family or even go on holiday somewhere, I would take an anti-depressant. None of this would be classed as depression (except SAD), but that it is what I think!

What it must be like to have depression day in day out, week in week out, year in year out, I can only imagine. All I know is that even my three-month spell of it was indescribable

Optimism and Pessimism.

This is not medically based but a service using perspective on hopes and fears.Psychotic delusions can seem so real that it would take a miracle to shift them. Importantly therefore, it must be noted that drugs can be called 'miracle cures'. Indeed the change can seem so amazing that such cures are also called 'wonder drugs'. What is more, the transformation can take place literally 'overnight'. Sometimes it is just a matter of finding the right one although this can take some time.

It is often wondered by patients if certain types of medication are designed for certain sets of symptoms and also if, perhaps, that there may be some mysterious set of criteria that must govern such choices. Quite often however, the choice is random or else it may be thought that some experimentation is required to find the right drug or combination of drugs. Psychiatrists may also disagree about the relative effectiveness of different drugs and such views may also change over time.

Chemical treatments seem very often to contend with 'alternative' homeopathic remedies, E.G 'Wolf's Bane' for schizophrenia and 'Saint John's Wort' for depression. What are we to make of these alternatives?

It may be argued that they have acquired popularity because of the seeming intractability of psychiatric problems. Originally psychiatrists managed to only cure one third of patients, yet the same is still true today of the most 'advanced' drugs including Clozapine, Risperidone and Olanzipine. Doctors have isolated a combination of genes that may pre-dispose the patient to schizophrenic illness. Such treatments are still decades away, not surprisingly therefore people look for alternative approaches.

Most lay people seem to have got the impression both that the brain seems to be so complex that they will never fully understand it and also what is to the contrary the belief that neuro-science, genetics and bio-chemistry are achieving amazing things. Take for example the television programs made by Lord Winston on the workings of the brain. Many people seem both to be amazed and dismissive of modern medicine. Take for example the often-repeated statement that "they still cannot cure the common cold!" How does such scepticism relate to psychiatry?

It is also well known that doctors can get it wrong and also judge their proximity of solutions to medical problems. In psychiatry for example, the introduction of the drug Clozapine caused the destruction of Leucocytes (or white blood cells), vital to the body's immune system. This caused the death of a number of patients. This drug is still widely used but requires a frequent blood test to protect the patient. There are also more significant examples.

The great hope for many sufferers seems to me to be, that genetic science will make a breakthrough and it has been mooted that this may be the potential cure for all known diseases. This was largely the result of the use of the retro virus which was used invade the cells of the body (where genes are located) to effect a cure. It worked but accidentally set off the gene that causes cancer of the blood. A follow up experiment at the University of Pennsylvania also caused the death of a volunteer. It is thought by some, according to the BBC's 'Horizon' programme, that genetic cures are in fact nowhere nearer than they were ten years ago.

So are we entitled to be more pessimistic or optimistic about the possibility of curing our psychiatric problems? There is certainly a perception of both. This however, is not the point of the account, and in any case, I am not qualified to answer it. The important point is that it is necessary to be optimistic. It took years to find the right drug and even the same drug may have to be tried a number of times before it works. For all the above posturings by the anti-psychiatry movement and alternative treatments etc., the medicines in use can really 'work wonders' and 'achieve miracles', as they have done for me.

Depression and stress may have been the triggers for my Schizophrenia.

Language and Stigma

In order to gauge the problem of the stigma of mental illness it is necessary to see how many words and phrases, heavily used by the media stigmatising those with the illness. The results are quite surprising. There are at least fifty-two such words and phrases. These are:

Loony, loopy, round-the-bend, round-the-twist, crazy, crackers, off your rocker, off your trolley, nuts, not a full shilling, not a full pound, not all there, daft, screw loose, mad-as-a-hatter, mad-as-a- march-hare, not a full deck, zany, mental, cranky, deranged, raving, loco, out of your mind, off your head, dotty, potty, batty, cuckoo, one sandwich short of a picnic, balmy, bonkers, bananas, screwy, insane, disturbed, unhinged, barking, fruit cake, nut case, head case, flipped, snapped, wacko, lost it, not right, loosing your marbles, mental, funny, abnormal, mad and non compus mentus.

These words are not the only labels, but they also further infect other everyday notions and as such, form a separate group of terms. Examples of this include the phrases "sick joke", "insane laughter", "ranting and raving", "insanely jealous", "screwed up", "hopping mad", "cracked up", "madly in love", "method to your madness", "mad axe-man", "mad scientist", "frayed ends of sanity", "mad driver", "it's a crazy world", "the lunatics are running the asylum", "acting like a maniac", "daft as a brush" and "tipped over the edge". Fifteen such further phrases in all.

These words and phrases are reinforced by a number of other terminological considerations: doctors are referred to as 'shrinks' and hospitals as the 'loony bin', 'nut house', 'funny farm', 'bedlam' or 'mad house', being run by the infamous 'men in white coats.' Such people are 'committed' rather than 'admitted' and 'certified' rather 'diagnosed.' This latter aspect is also exemplified in the 1960`s song "There coming to take me away, Ha!" All this, when the existence of medical terminology was meant to dispel the stigma. We shall examine all these groups of terms and their origins later.

In relation to the popular definition of mental illness and the stigma of being mentally ill, a number of further considerations seem also to be worth noting here. These relate to the common misuse of the following words and phrases referring to mental illness: 'dual' or 'split' personality for schizophrenia, 'madness' or 'insanity' for mental illness, and 'psychopathic' for psychotic. These words seem to be at the root of much of the stigma experienced by people with mental illness.

In the case of the first instance, the notion that schizophrenia is a dual personality, the origin of this example appears to be the story of 'Jekyll and Hyde'. Notwithstanding the fact that there exists something else called 'multiple personality disorder', the prefix 'Schizo' signifies to most people a 'divide', 'split', or 'schism' within the self, hence suggests the common misperception of schizophrenia noted here.

The 'Jekyll and Hyde' story, connects well with those cases heavily reported in the media, where schizophrenics have been violent towards themselves or other people. This connection has also been used in a number of well known films including Alfred Hitchcock's 'Psycho', and 'The Shining' starring Jack Nicholson. Here the central character is a knife-wielding 'maniac', or 'mad axe-man' respectively. The protagonist is 'insane' or 'mad' rather than 'ill', and is 'psychopathic' rather than 'psychotic.'

Origins.

The origins of much of the present stigma of having a mental illness, appear to lie in the Victorian period. To illustrate this it is useful to explore some of the of the words used to describe the mentally ill – in particular the word 'lunatic' and the phrase 'cracked up.'

The first derives from the days of padded cells and straight jackets. The second is a disparaging term for a nervous breakdown deriving from the Victorian ethic of self-help and self-reliance. The word 'lunatic' conjures up images of mad people out of control, needing restraint, and confinement in an asylum. Underlying this social exclusion and physical confinement, is the fear that mad people may turn violent. This is a premise heavily influenced by continual reports in the media of acts of violence by schizophrenics towards themselves or others – all of which helps conjure up the 'Hannibal Lecter' image of the mentally ill. Such films and reports reinforce negative connotations of the word 'lunatic.'

The other image of mental illness is that such people have 'cracked up' under pressure. Such individuals are said to have 'lost it' (it referring to their sanity) and are seen as weak compared to those who can cope with life. To 'crack up' is not a socially acceptable reaction and such people 'ought to pull themselves together' or 'grin and bear it.'

Is it also 'cowardly' to commit suicide? People seem to think this is the 'easy' way out and that such people cannot 'face up' to their problems. People have much the same attitude to alcoholism. Some would perhaps argue that suicide is not easy but actually the opposite. However, we rarely see the hero or heroine in films or the media cast as courageous and heroic for surviving schizophrenia etc. or commended on the suicide?

It is these notions i.e. of the existence of 'lunatics' and that some people 'loose it ' and 'crack up', which seem to have contributed to what Foucault calls 'the great confinement' (in asylums) that occurred during modern times. These notions are thus at the root of the stigma experienced by people who have schizophrenia or manic depression.

Meanings.

It is interesting to note the origin and meaning of those stigmatising words and phrases which label schizophrenia and manic depression. Sarah Maitland in an article in Openmind suggested we try to reclaim these terms. The origins of these words fall into four basic categories. First is the technical source, second are those words and phrases coined in popular parlance, third are words and phrases which are literary in origin and finally words and phrases which are simply slang in origin. We shall briefly examine each in turn; constraints of space however prevent an exhaustive enquiry.

The first group includes words such 'lunatic', 'manic', 'madness', 'non compus mentis' and 'insane'. 'Lunatic' for example is Roman/Latin in origin. The Romans believed (in the way modern Astrologers do) that the phases of the moon influenced behaviour, including behavioural abnormalities. It is curious that the word has survived so long given it's meaning. 'Insane' is equally curious as it merely signifies the absence of something and does not denote any positive characteristics. 'Non compus mentis' seems to imply that there is some kind of deficiency, which in popular parlance carries a stigma because it implies non-competence.

The second group are not technical words but are still used in standard English. These include 'zany', 'raving', 'crazy', 'mental' and 'deranged'. Some of these words can be used in a non-derogatory way but only the word 'mental' directly relates to the problems experienced by psychiatric patients (a point to which I shall return). The word 'bedlam', derived from the Victorian asylum 'Bethlem', is still used in common language to mean 'a state of uproar and confusion' despite the fact that most modern hospitals are in fact quiet and restful. 'Deranged' and 'raving' meanwhile, are very derogatory terms.

The third group are words that have acquired authority through their appearance in great works of Literature. Lewis Carrol's 'Alice in Wonderland' is a good example as it contains the 'Mad hatter's tea party'. The phrases appearing therein of 'Mad-as-a-hatter' and 'mad-as-a-March-Hare' have passed into language. The first is curious since the Victorians believed that the Mercury used in the rim of a top hat helping weigh it down was responsible for driving the people who made them mad! The second phrase refers to the way Hares gad about in March's rutting season. This does look quite manic. We have already noted the story of Jekyll and Hyde.

The final group; slang words, is the largest and falls into two sub categories: ones that contain some insight and ones that do not. Being 'nuts' relates directly to mental problems since your 'nut' is a slang word for the head, thus it refers to some problem with it. Other slang terms are more oblique but contain the same kernel of meaning. Having a 'screw loose' for example implies there is something wrong and in need of fixing. Other slang terms (ones which fall into the secondary category above) in contrast, are devoid of meaning. These include 'potty', 'dotty', 'batty', 'balmy', bonkers etc.

It may be objected, that in normal parlance these words can also be used in a jocular way. Even the word 'shrink' can be harmlessly used to refer to psychiatrists in the way people refer to medical doctors as 'quacks'. Nevertheless there is a social stigma relating to mental illness sometimes through the corruption of technical terms. This is how it is expressed. It is instructive to consider an example.

Many of the words used in popular and curiously also in technical parlance lend themselves to meanings which are stigmatising. Consider for example the transmutation of the phrase 'lunatic asylum' into 'loony bin.' In the end it would be helpful if we stopped employing even such quasi-technical terms as 'insane' and referred instead only to the more medical sounding referents such as 'mental illness' or 'psychiatric problem' and of 'lunatic asylums' as 'psychiatric hospitals.'

The use of 'politically correct' language has been instrumental in combating other types of prejudice such as racism (blacks as 'wogs'), homophobias (gays as 'benders' and lesbians as 'dykes') and also gender neutral language. It would therefore also be of key importance in the area of mental health promotion. The employment of such terms in the media (as has been done in other areas of social life) is vital in raising awareness. Curiously however the terminology of mental health stigma is the one major aspect of social life that has yet to be reformed in the media. Some meanings perpetuate ignorance other contain insight – we shall examine these problems later.

Engagement with Madness

The layman has historically had a five-fold engagement with madness; there has been both the fascination and the fear of madness, comedy and ridicule, and finally hostility. It is worth exploring both attitudes to the extent they might shed some light on (some of) the historical origins of the stigma.

Part of the fascination with madness lies in the popular myth referring to mental illness, that genius is 'touched' by madness. In many ways this seems to be how society has coped with those in it's midst, who are capable of turning what everyone thinks upside down. Thus madness is a category imposed on some by others as a means of social control. Take for example the 'mad philosopher' Friedrich Nietzsche who was imprisoned in a late nineteenth century asylum, or the abuses of psychiatry in the former Soviet Union - the way dissidents like the physicist Anatolie Sheransky were treated. Van Gogh Cut his ear off.

The second aspect of the fascination with madness lies in the notion that the mad person has somehow escaped the strain of the responsibilities and pressures of modern life. The fear of madness begins with it's misrepresentation by the media and in literature such as 'Jekyll and Hyde'. What is so terrifying about these tales and their modern day equivalents such as 'Hannibal Lecter' is that they try and get inside the mind of the mentally ill as something abnormal. The patient is therefore exploited for the shock value with little of the appropriate medical context involved. This also creates a further aspect of fascination.

Thus fascination and fear (shock value) have historically resulted in an insatiable curiosity about madness. Thus in Victorian times, people were drawn to lunatic asylums (like 'Bethlem') to see for themselves what madness is. Although it was never hospital policy to promote this, patients were put on show to the general public, laughed at and mocked for their 'unusual' behaviour and 'absurd' delusional ideas. This I think is one origin of the stigma of mental illness resulting in the view that madness is comical and / or ridiculous.

Other more recent examples of the (mis-) perception that madness is comical can be found in the 'Inspector Cleauceau' comedies were the madman 'Dreyfuss' is incarcerated in a padded cell babbling about the former with a nervous twitch! In the second case above of the perception of madness as ridiculous, we can find a more recent example in Bram Stoker's 'Dracula' were the character 'Renfield' is likewise incarcerated in an asylum whose governor mockingly asks him "oh!, so you think you are God I suppose?"

More recent examples of this kind of comedy and ridicule can be found in the 1960's song: "there coming to take me away ha! Ha!" Another may be found in the character of Doctor Silverman in Terminator 2 who laughs at the notional delusions of the principle protagonist Sarah Conner – that a robot from the future is trying to kill her and at the fact that it looks human so that there is no evidence to the contrary. The same character in the first Terminator movie also declares mockingly that the character Reece is "in technical terms he's a loon!"

The establishment of asylums had an unintended consequence – it led to the perception that there was 'something wrong' with the inhabitants. They became known as the 'funny farm' or 'loony bin' and the word 'Bedlam' passed into language. Doctors, instead of transforming the understanding of 'madness' into 'mental illness became infamous as the 'men in white coats.' The underlying mis-perception here, is that there is something 'abnormal' about the mental y ill which has resulted in both hostility and stigma towards madness.

The story does not end here however. It is thus left to ask: why does this aspect of the stigma exist? One reason is that, simply, people have something to gain by affirming their 'normality' in this respect: it allows people to demonstrate their 'soundness' by being able to say "well I'm not like that." This infers a mark of superiority while the mentally ill are implied to be deficient, abnormal or even unnatural and hence some of the origins of the stigma. These attitudes and reactions have created myths and ignorance about mental illness – we shall examine this problems later.

Confinement.

Foucault famously called the asylums the great confinement. This essay focuses on exclusion and confinement. This I think is the possibly the most important and dangerous aspect of the stigma and should therefore be outlined in more detail than in my earlier account. Concentration in asylums is easy to stigmatise.

The language of the spatial segregation of the mentally ill in asylums can reinforce the social exclusion of schizophrenics in particular as it gives rise to the popular myth that lunatics need separating and locking up. This is reinforced by the popular notion such places are like bedlam requiring restraints, padded cells and straight jackets.

Socially to the mentally ill exclusion from 'normal' society in such places may seem like a social or even a moral prison. These fears on the part of the mentally ill about others attitudes towards them (hostility) and the fear, on the part of the community, of the mentally ill (who may be violent) mean that the occasional walls around hospitals function as a psychological security barrier for people on both sides. Such walls become a physical symbol and the incarnation of this divide else the occasional remoteness of hospital buildings help to institutionalise the spatial separation of the mentally ill by creating a self enclosed little world with little 'outside contact.'

The lack of contact with such places and the outside world has created a number of myths and notions about such places. They became known as the 'funny farm', 'loony bin', 'bedlam' or 'lunatic asylum.' Doctors became known as the 'men in white coats' and as one writer in 'Breakthrough' pointed out that in the popular perception is that people would disappear into such places and never be heard of again. The most abiding media image is that such places are ones of confinement.

This can be found in the asylums in popular films such as 'Hannibal Lecter' and 'Terminator 2'. Meanwhile a recent headline in 'The Sun' newspaper, with reference to a famous boxer, declared 'Bonkers Bruno Locked up!' The reason for this abiding image is not just the sensationalism of Hollywood films but is continually reinforced by reports in the media of cases where schizophrenics have been violent towards themselves or other people. The most famous case of this which received massive media coverage perhaps is that of the 'Yorkshire Ripper' Peter Sutcliff who has been detained in Broadmoor high security hospital. Sometimes the way this is presented the impression created would seem to be that there is little difference between a Schizophrenic and a Psychopath – a connection we noted first made in R. L. Stevenson's 'Jekyll and Hyde'.

The spatial divide infects the language we use to describe this state of affairs: we speak of people being 'out there' in a hostile community (and of hospital as 'in here'). The allusion to the spatial confinement of the mentally ill is also evident from a number of other unconsciously used phases such as when people are referred to as being 'taken away' or 'carted off' to the loony bin – and of people being 'committed' instead of 'admitted' . People even talk of people 'escaping' from hospital and there are the repeated headlines such as "nutters on the loose.". Take for example the song "they are coming to take me away Ha Ha!" The popular image of being locked up is not helped by the notion of compulsory confinement implicit in the legal power of a section and ultimately by the existence of locked wards and secure hospitals.

An example of this sort of thinking can even be found to a small extent in the official government policy strategy of care 'in' the community. This creates the impression that care was previously somehow outside of the 'wider society' an allusion which recurs in the so named government 'social exclusion unit' who area of competence includes mental health. Perhaps even the current existence of housing associations providing 'sheltered accommodation' for mentally ill people has tended to reinforce the related and older (but still popular) notion that hospitals are still a 'refuge' or 'asylum' from the society which in another sense might imply that such places are elsewhere.

Much then depends on awareness of the language we use to describe such places. We now talk of being 'sectioned' instead of 'committed.' The trouble here is that the word implies an element of compulsion which could give the wrong impression. 'Admitted' is by far and away the best term possible. The notions of confinement serve to further create and reinforce the social divide which this language expresses.

In sum the notions of psychiatric hospitals as places where we lock up lunatics and various terms which create this impression outlined above are best avoided since where we have separate groups without social interaction the various myths and stigma surrounding mental illness can only be reinforced in the ways outlined above. Politically correct language, (particularly in terms of notions of confinement as outlined above) is again of key importance here. Care in the community on this account, should go a long way to undoing the stigma of mental illness in this respect due to the isolation of psychiatric hospitals certainly being one source of ignorance about mental health. (a notion very closely connected to mental health stigma which we shall examine shortly).

Obviously the reality of being admitted is very much the reverse to the Hollywood and media image. Many admissions are voluntary and in my own experience I have seen very few examples where some kind of force or compulsion has been necessary. I think that this aspect of stigma is so out of touch with hospital that this last point does not even need underlining.

Ignorance and Prejudice.

Any attempt at the reform of attitudes towards mental health, namely the stigma, to many seems a deceptively simple task. All that needs to be done is to combat people's ignorance so that, as the reasoning suggests, is to talk about and to educate. Ignorance; which I think is the key concept in this view, is unconsciously used by people and as with the notion of prejudice, is a more complicated notion to deploy.

If at one level it seems intuitively correct to call the stigma of mental health a 'prejudice', at another level it could be (and often is) called 'ignorance'. 'Ignorance' is conventionally defined as a lack of knowledge and assuming we think of it this way, education seems the appropriate response. Reform of language too by calling it 'mental illness' instead of 'madness' for example, could it was hoped change attitudes and make people more aware.

At another level ignorance could be defined and interpreted differently. It implies that something is ignored. Ironically to ignore something in this way once it is pointed out to us, could be seen as even more ignorant (i.e. we can ignore the fact that we are ignorant). This use of the word however is also subject to the same definition (that we are ignoring something), the original problem therefore remains. Thus if we point out that someone is ignorant they would probably say "well I don't care!" The question thus then becomes "why do people ignore such things?"

Crucially this is because they already have an attitude which conflicts with the issue, about which there is (to others) a question. So perhaps the issue is not about ignorance at whatever level, but the underlying attitude and prejudice?

The equation is that of ignorance and cultural beliefs so that mental health prejudice serves to advantage some in society at the expense of others. It allows some people to gain a sense of superiority through their self-proclaimed and normatively charged 'toughness' while the 'weak' are stigmatised. So ignorance appears not so much as a deficit of knowledge but rather also as a social attitude to life.

A number of famous quotes are now of direct relevance here, where the words 'ignorance' and 'reason' crop up again and again;

"The prejudices of ignorance are more easily removed than the prejudices of interest; the first are blindly adopted, the second wilfully preferred."
-George Bancroft

"Prejudice is never easy unless it can pass itself off for reason."
-William Hazlitt

"A prejudiced person will almost certainly claim

that he has sufficient warrant for his views."
-Gordon W. Allport

People in the know, such as nurses and social workers, will refer to the stigma of mental health dismissively and say "oh that's just ignorance." In fact this is a problematic and difficult thing to say as the ignorance derives from beliefs about life. The 'ignorance' here is wilful and contrary to being unaware of their actions, people know what they are doing in creating a stigma. Society seems to need a 'whipping boy' and to pick on the vulnerable. Some further quotes are very relevant:

"Opinions founded on prejudice are always sustained with the greatest violence".
-Francis Jeffrey

"Nothing in the world is more dangerous than a sincere ignorance and conscientious stupidity."
Author: Martin Luther King, Jr.

"Nothing is more terrible than ignorance in action."
Author: Johann Wolfgang von Goethe

The stigma of mental illness can be compared in this respect, to the other areas of social life such as racism, homophobia and the sub-ordination of women. Racists and the like are not ignorant to the hurt and fear they cause to other people. Like everybody else they have a moral sensibility, its just that they 'ignore' it. Such people are to some extent choosing to behave in this way and so can be held responsible. The law for example, makes it illegal to discriminate against people on the grounds of race, gender, sexuality and psychiatric history in terms of employment and any other form of social activity. 'Ignorantia legis haut non excusat' -ignorance of the law is no excuse in court!

The aspect of ignorance seems apparent from the nature of the stigma and the language. Most people cannot distinguish between a psychologist and a psychiatrist, between mental health and mentally handicapped and between schizophrenia and a split personality. This does not bode well for the medical semantic emphasis on the notions of mental illness and mental health coined instead of madness, and of hospitals instead of asylums.

Criticism of attitudes towards mental illness then strike at the heart of the cultural beliefs that Burke argued were pervasive features of social life, namely at the rough tough 'stiff upper lip' required to face life's difficulties and over come them. This Victorian work ethic of self help and self reliance and is ultimately part of the British character and national identity. Perhaps attitudes like these are so deeply rooted in our culture that the task of reform seems almost impossible?

This leads directly to consideration of a related notion, as William Hazlitt famously said "prejudice is the child of ignorance." Perhaps we should be given the option of studying some Psychiatry at school. Even amongst educated professional people today however, there is still a stigma about seeing a 'shrink'. The media must also play a lead educational role here in changing the image of madness; films such as 'A Beautiful Mind' are exemplary because as it portrayed a schizophrenic as a high achiever.

Racism, gender issues etc. have already attracted a lot of academic (and educational) attention yet some of this does not give cause for optimism about mental health stigma. Take for instance the current charge of 'institutional racism' levelled by the Steven Lawrence enquiry, the recent electoral successes by the British National Party in Oldham and the sociological scepticism about the idea of the 'new man', which has been called a modern myth given that many working women also have the sole burden of house work, child care etc. Prejudice seems 'endemic' in many areas of social life.

Why is there a stigma?

The stigma of mental illness arises from the belief or prejudice that men are suppose to be tough and able to overcome life's difficulties or whatever life throws at them. The general attitude is expressed by popular sayings such as "life is hard" and "life is not a bowl of cherries." The tough minded attitude seems to be the origin of the stigma of mental illness. It opens the way for derision of those who cannot cope as weak and incapable, it stigmatises those in need of help. If you are depressed you "just have to get on with it" and "pull yourself together." Ultimately "you should not need help" as in the end, "it is up to you to help yourself." There is little understanding or sympathy, in some peoples view, of mental health and especially depression as an illness. Indeed it challenges the whole concept of a more humane approach to mental illness.

If the opinion is handed down that this is a medical problem and is refused by scepticism in society because of its historic cultural inheritance, then the result is ignorance and prejudice. If on the other hand, the reaction is that this diagnosis (to some extent), is persuasive and makes some kind of sense, then people will think of it as a legitimate medical problem. This may be especially true if for example, medication prevents a persons suicide many people may be then sympathetic to the need for medical help. The danger is that it may also create the impression that they are weak or "taking the easy way out" or even that "they don't deserve any help." Most people will be torn between both extremes. This to me opens up questions about people having an interest in promoting stigma in this sense and also the possibility of changing attitudes based on self interest.

We may call the view we are examining "enlightened." Prejudice in contrast is often "dark" and clouds our understanding. It is to be criticised in the area of mental health through coming to know what the object of the prejudice is, i.e. if we work with people with a mental illness then we will become sympathetic and try to help them. From this perspective, prejudice is not only "blind" and insensitive but is cruel and "victimises" the social group involved. At the limit we cannot really "know" the problems of depression and schizophrenia unless we have had it ourselves, but we cannot fail to see someone "going through" this and not react to it. We want to help but don't know how. Medication is the most direct approach possible when faced with this dilemma.

But there is a problem. As we have said people will be torn between sympathy and blame even in the case of suicide. It is thought to be both selfish and stupid, though if we know the person involved we may be sympathetic and perhaps blame ourselves that we did not do enough to prevent it. We talk of people being "pushed to the limit". The problem is that others go through the same experience but do not "resort to killing them selves." The consensus for some is that "this is a matter of private judgement" and perhaps not of public concern. Others think that we must do everything possible to "prevent this sort of thing." Nowadays this includes medical treatment.

It may be that some people with the same amount of stress or who have gone through the same experiences did not kill themselves. They are seen as stronger and so the prejudice arises. It is difficult to say anything conclusive and often the subject is never discussed. I think most people would say it is wrong, but not with absolute certainty. It is seen as the extreme example. The whole issue is "difficult", though some brave people have 'fixed' negative views on the subject. Thus if others want to ask for medical help it would be denied them. Those who do are stigmatised and not considered as behaving acceptably. At this point they are labelled as "weak" and "immoral" and so the stigma begins. They can be used as examples to show how "tough" the others are. This is the right attitude to life and is reflected in culture and human society which presents all kinds of like challenges that must be "faced up to". Those who do not are 'cowards' by not "confronting" the "way the world is." If they kill themselves, then "that is up to them" but they "will get no sympathy from me".

Castigating the whole idea of mental health in this way leads to the view that people with depression are not facing up to their problems. If others survive experiences like divorce, domestic violence, unemployment or warfare so they must be weak or incapable. Here we get the view that I am "better" than them because I am "stronger". This is to be admired and moralised into a virtue and principle. It is something to which we aspire. It serves a world view in which people who do cope, have an esteemed position. Those who do not are derided as having, in some sense, "failed". Those who succeed in "overcoming their problems" have a social status. The strong label themselves in accordance with their reasoning, but confront a perceived disputing problem with respect to their values. To acquire this status in the eyes of other people and allay feelings of guilt, they must conform and perhaps are afraid not to. This prevents seeking help and makes us "keep our feelings quiet".

It is in the interests of people in society that they attain this self esteem. We conform because of how other people might see us and the pressures of praise and blame. But where we deal with an interest in promoting these beliefs, say for the perceived good of the society and the individual, we run up against the problem that where an interest is involved, the prejudice is more difficult to eradicate. How far can we change such a view of the social interest?

The stigma of mental health thus has a psychological dimension. We have noted that the stigma of not being able to cope with depression - to pull oneself together and grin and bear it – is cultural – having a stiff upper lip - but this can also be reduced to psychology. This attitude could be derived from our notion of masculinity – men are not suppose to show their feelings and worst of all break down and cry. Such behaviour is conversely the province of femininity – though there seems to be potential improvement in this aspect of the stigma associated with the 'new man'.

Also relevant under fear is the notion that mental health problems are things that anyone can get and thus it is necessary to proclaim ones normality in this respect. This drives at an individual level to create a stigma about abnormality. Stress and depression are thought to make people crack up under pressure if subject to enough of this however strong they think they are. The result is a 'nervous breakdown.' This challenges the theory that it is only people who can't cope that suffer this. Against the enlightened and humane view of mental health is societies view of it as an abnormality.

It allows people to demonstrate their "soundness" by being able to say if the enlightened view is true "well I'm not like that." This infers a mark of superiority while the mentally ill are thought to be abnormal or even (like the prejudice over sexuality) unnatural. There is the perceived conflict of interests. Some people thus begin to have an in interest in promoting this image because it challenges cherished notions of nature and social life. They have succeeded where others have failed but opposing this is the view that had the circumstances been different the outcome may not have been the same. Do they simply have an interest here because they are stronger?

Combating the language of stigma.

Reform of mental health stigma has mainly been opposed, on the basis of scientific understanding, the notions of 'mental health' and 'mental illness' to 'madness'. Despite some positive media images to the contrary, the language of being 'off your rocker' and 'round the twist' prevails in the media and in everyday speech at a subconscious level. Much more needs to be done however through an examination of the language of the stigma.

'Madness' in point of fact is an example of what is a called an umbrella term or Lewis Carroll called a 'Portmanteau Word', in that it tries to put some very different things into the same box. I suspect that this is because society has had a tendency to simply label any behaviour which it does not understand in the same way. Thus manias, melancholia, delusions, paranoia, hallucinations, simple schizophrenia, hebephrenia, catatonia, schizo-affective disorder, bi-polar, hypo-manic, hyper-manic, hearing voices etc.' have been so grouped together. But what does this 'madness' mean other than the loss of reason?

Thus similar such words tend to be defined in a purely negative way: it is abnormal, insane, unusual, non-sensical, non-compus mentis, deficient, deranged and not rational. i.e. people are thought to have 'lost their minds'. The negative definitional aspect of madness can also be found in a number of popularly used slang expressions such as 'not all there', 'not right', 'not a full shilling', 'not a full deck', 'one sandwich short of a picnic' etc. But again what is all this negative talk really about?

This to me suggests a strategy to combat mental health stigma on an everyday level. All words are defined by reference to other words. If we press someone further to explain what is meant by "balmy" or "bonkers" etc, often we find that in the popular mind no further definition is available beyond referring back to another such word in the slang vocabulary e.g. "deranged", "cranky", "crackers" etc. I think underlying the use of such labels is the intuition that people do not really know what these words mean. This can be readily exposed.

Often in every day terms, madness can be seen as a coping mechanism for acute stresses in life that can find no other outlet. Consider for example how often the phrase "you'll drive me mad!" is said on an every day level. Deployment of this notion should also attempt at removing some of the social stigma of the illness It coincides with the current psychological theory that stress can cause psychoses. Other such phrases here include being "tipped over the edge", "the frayed ends of sanity" and "driven round the bend."

Other words linked to the stigma have different connotations. In particular the notions of being 'locked up', 'taken away' or 'carted off.' Foucault famously picked up on this and defined the birth of the asylum "the great confinement." Most people have probably heard of 'care in the community' and so reference to this in reply to such statements might help combat the image of mental illness. I also believe it is necessary to also stop talking about being 'sectioned' because it sounds too much like the old word 'committed.'

Words can then be weapons, a careful consideration therefore of the language of the stigma and the elements and degree of insight such usage involves could provide a useful armoury in the battle to transform attitudes to mental health. Thus the word 'mental' has some insight as it refers to the mind, having a 'screw loose' meanwhile implies that something is in need of fixing, thus can be compared to the word 'batty' or 'potty', both containing little idea of what is being talked about.

The most direct approach in such a war of words and political correctness perhaps, is to turn the language of the stigma against it's users to question what he or she think they know about it, thus exposing the ignorance of his or her notions. Political correctness is the key.

Care in the community

Was 'Care in the community' just another attempt to save money by selling off hospitals without regard to the best possible arrangements for the patients and medical staff? Was it because the drugs were any better, allowing less need for supervision and support? The answer as far as anti-psychotics are concerned is no. They only cure 33% of patients, yet the majority are now discharged into the community. In the case of the former question, the answer is also no, as it embraces some of the more difficult social and political questions central to Margaret Thacther's own brand of conservative ideology.

'Care in the community' had a seeming dubious philosophical basis for it's pioneer Margaret Thatcher, who famously argued that there is no such thing as society. This fact is more interesting in the context of the dissolution of communities and it's replacement by individualism. In relating with other people, things become more anonymous creating less scope for social contact. The reason the Victorians built these places in the first instance was, in contrast, to foster a sense of community. Margaret Thatcher also argued for Victorian values and self help which also seems to be relevant to her mental health policies

Institutionalisation and dependency are the product of hospitalisation. Being in the community in contrast, means taking responsibility for ones own life and making one's own decisions and choices without someone to rely on. Such freedom is now seen as part of our conception of human dignity and also has a philosophical bases. Was this affronted by the old system of asylum? Did it sometimes feel like a prison or that society did not want them? Do people feel included in the community and excluded in hospital? Therefore is 'Care in the community' the answer here?

The hope is that, as Michel Oakeshott argued; "freedom is something we have learned to enjoy." This would bode well for mental health. However other contemporary conservative philosophers like Roger Scruton argue that such "freedom, is one of man's deepest felt anxieties" and what is required instead, is a sense of community. This contradicts the potential therapeutic content of Oakeshott's view of freedom. Would the mentally ill have to face anomie, in addition to their other problems?

Material dependency is another aspect of life that has been targeted with regards to mental health matters. Being able to work and support oneself is not only rewarding in that it gives one self a sense of achievement, not to mention a sense of 'normality' (whatever that is!). Thus we have sheltered workshops, disabled training colleges like the one at Finchale in Durham, positive discrimination and disability employment advisors etc. The flip side of this view of work is that, as Marxists have argued for 150 years, it creates alienation which could also create further problems of the mentally ill.

Perhaps the most serious critique of the notion of 'Care in the community' is of that provided by the left wing psychiatrist R.D. Laing. Laing is famous as the psychiatrist who thought that an irrational world was responsible for driving people mad. The old term for hospital: 'asylum', was a refuge away from other people and society. In the current context of psychological theories on mental health, stress can cause psychiatric illness. Life in general and work in particular can be very stressful, as can the stigma surrounding 'lunatics.' 'Care in the community' exposes the patient to all of this.

Does this policy also dispel the stigma attached to 'hospitals?' Certainly, they now cannot be labelled loony bin, funny farm, nut house etc. However these notions of 'loony', being a bit 'funny' and being 'nuts' are still general and popular. In some respect, hospitals seem to have reinforced the stigma. Hostility on part of the community and the media, has been effected by stories highlighting mistakes made by doctors where released patients have committed murders and other crimes under the 'care in the community' policy. Former health secretary Frank Dobson came in for a good deal of criticism on this issue.

The experience of Waddington Street has generally been positive and seems to show that 'Care in the community', for all it's philosophical problems, has been a good thing. You still cannot go down the pub and say your schizophrenic! However we can meet up at such places with other people (including people who are not ill at mental health day centres) and still enjoy a full social life. Things are not perfect, for instance local yobs come and put our windows out. Then again nothing is perfect. All in all I like being 'out' of hospital even if that does not mean I am altogether 'in' the community.

Interestingly then it can be argued that 'Care in the community' was misconceived and did not take into account the social stigma and other problems confronting the mentally ill 'out there' in the community. I feel the experience in my case has been mixed, it is interesting to reflect on the supposed reasons for this.

Of course, 'hospitalisation' had its down side as well: dependency, institutionalisation and what Foucault famously called the 'great confinement' imposed by a 'carcereal society.' After years of criticising all this, do we now seem any more happier with the alternative to being in society?

Although of course we now have more 'individual freedom', the original point of the program in terms of what is called greater self-determination (i.e. new education or employment opportunities, money to go shopping, setting our own menu, to live where and go anywhere we like, perhaps nearer our families etc), we still often seem to miss the social contact and the supportive environment offered by group living in a hospital community.

This was always a problem for the philosophy behind the 'Care in the community' program for some of the conservatives who pioneered it. Margaret Thatcher at the same time famously said there was no such thing as society!! But seriously this is, in fact, the real crux of the problem with the policy. Without society (if people believe this), there may be atomism and anomie plus the fact that the 'opportunity' of having to work may bring alienation. All of this on top of mental health problems.

On the positive side of this philosophy, the so called 'freedom of the individual' the Thatcherite policy envisaged, has it seems for many people today, replaced the importance of being a part of the community. Everybody is free to enjoy 'doing their own thing' (regardless of what the community or society thinks). If we really do enjoy this freedom of choice, it may be that social life has improved, at least in these respects. Being 'in the real world' therefore may not be such a bad place after all. On the whole I do quite like it. To this extent I find that this 'self-determination' can be quite empowering. But were these grand words and high ideals also just a rather rosy picture of the social life out there?

There are the obvious problems, like crime, associated with the loss of community feeling.

However I feel the main problem is that exposing people to community brings us into contact with all kinds of social problems. A look at how a 'community' can act should reflect this. It is ridden by conflicts and prejudices which the mentally ill must also live with in addition to their own problems.

Thus even 'village life' often works to exclude people they, for any reason, do not like. Thus people in small villages often do not seem to like and sometimes wish to exclude 'incomers.' I am from one myself and there maybe some real examples of community ignorances and myths here. Thus the new growth of 'commuter villages' creates a lot of social conflict: 'City folk' for example, supposedly, see country life as insular, parochial, even semi-feudal in much the same way as northerners think southerners are 'less friendly.' Social life was never perfect and is ridden by conflicts of all kinds, the problem of stigma is a just a further example of how imperfect it can be (it is this kind of ignorance on the part of people which creates the stigma anyway).

I also sometimes have some real doubts about the philosophy supporting 'Care in the community' through the problems we have been discussing. Living in any 'institution' like a school, hospital or university campus, does create a group context. Modern mass society however is not such a small scale entity and probably never was. Think, for example, of the dislike (not to mention fear) rural villagers (notionally) seem to have of living in anonymous big cities like London, where "nobody knows anybody, not even their neighbours…" What is called anomie is for many people is often a pervasive belief and a real experience.

If the problem for mental health policy is that perhaps society is now actually more anonymous than a hospital community there may be other difficulties to the point about anomie. To be honest, I think most of this description can be very stereotypical even nowadays: thus we all still seem to enjoy watching 'Neighbours' and 'Emmerdale'. This may point to the current existence of community feeling. Thus one can still be a husband, wife, mother, neighbour and friend in spite of all this notional 'loss' in the idea of community.

Surely therefore our family and local friendships are what matter most, and irrespective of an 'anonymous mass society' which, at this level probably is largely composed of many 'other people' who we do not really know well or at all. But how can we think society in some form, as Thatcher argued, does not exist?

What does worry me though, if there is such a strong psychological need for community on the part of individuals then why have we lost the idea at all and claim there is no such thing? Would we not form a general or 'organic' community if we really did want one? Maybe life without it, for most people, is not so bad after all?

For the mentally ill this 'need' for community supports the reality of the problem (of integrating into the society we have been describing) and could be a real extra problem for the mentally ill already living in the 'big, bad world.' On the other hand the need could lead us to live in 'Coronation Street' in order to make social contact with others needing the same thing.

Yet still there is often still the need for social support: my local mental health day centre on Waddington Street in Durham, is itself such a small scale group which is why it seems to work for us as a community (within a town context). Like the regulars who 'go down the local' the atmosphere is friendly and relaxed. Simply having a place like this to go, like a sports club, light opera group or the local boozer as do others, is enough for me. I do not really miss the idea of the whole of society being such a community group as long as I still have a local circle of friends.

In my case, I thought that coming 'out' of a hospital community was going to be a very big social change, but I believe people are very adaptable with the right support. To me, the experience of 'going into' hospital was more of a change than 'coming out' considering I was in there for a year! Maybe, although I am not sure about this, the 'security' of a 'hospital community' now seems in reality to have been just 'all in my head?' Institutionalisation is a real problem but, with help, we can 'get out there' and we can also maybe 'get a life', much the same as everyone else! despite all this taking some getting used to, not to mention courage. So I find myself, with some reservations, supporting the idea of 'Care in the community'.

Being under Section.

Paranoia often takes it's focus on people within the immediate vicinity thus people very often think that the neighbours are persecuting them. If this happens in hospital whilst locked in, it makes the experience even more frightening and intense. This however can be a very subtle and complex reaction which depends on a number of considerations that mutually reinforce one another. There are ten relevant points here:

1. The length of time for a tribunal hearing to be arranged in order to overturn the section, is ten weeks and then six months for an appeal. Is this deliberate to keep you in there?

2. It is also law now that patients must take their tablets. How would this be interpreted by the patient? Might it be a toxin or part of the regime of restraint and consignment? Being doped up all day might be taken to mean that they are giving you something so you are less capable of 'escaping'. Are they deliberately trying to institutionalise you? Will you be 'locked up' forever?

3. It is argued that the brain is so complex that the drugs used are only a little more effective than those used in the past. They also have horrendous side effects. Sometimes the drugs cause psychoses, some even claim that they have gone out and committed murders whilst under the

influence of 'medicines'. All the more reason for paranoia?

4. Furthermore, what you often do not get to hear about is the anti-psychiatry movement. They see the psychiatric institution as an infringement of freedom, for example they see suicide as a civil right. Thinking of it in this way seems to be a further focus of paranoia as it criticises the 'help' you receive.

5. Some treatments like ECT are extremely frightening to contemplate, not to mention the still used practice of 'Leucotomy' better known as 'Lobotomy' which can cause brain damage and involves drilling holes in your skull which will not heal.

6. Being in hospital also distances you from friends and family. It is a strange environment full of strange people. Typically other people will display the same feeling of paranoia towards the nursing staff that you do, which may act to reinforce your own view of them.

7. Nurses run a system of observation and note taking which could be interpreted by a schizophrenic as spying or surveillance. What are these notes for and who else is going to read them? The same also applies for doctor's notes and questions. The freedom of information act might come in useful here? Are the stated reasons for the incarceration untrue?

8. Eventually you will have to be discharged. One reason for confinement is the danger you may pose to yourself. However, you may relapse when released and be out of reach of medical help. The thing is, this is also equally true of being in hospital where people also kill themselves, so why the section in the first place?

9. It may be however, that being in hospital enables you to gain some insight. There are others who think similar thoughts, some of whom will respond to treatment and be 'released' and 'discharged.' At the other extreme however, other patients will be violent and brought in or taken away in police cars. Do they bear you ill well also?

10. Then there is the stigma around the place in which you are 'sectioned.' This gets called the 'nut house', 'funny farm', 'loony bin' etc. Has society locked you in here for a reason – perhaps to be ridiculed or excluded?

Living in Sheltered Accommodation

Not like hospital, not like home. You do not have to share a room like in hospital and often there will be no staff during the night or at weekends. You are responsible for taking your own medication, for being able to call the 'out of hours' emergency line and to describe what is happening to you in a crisis. In this latter case, a project worker will come out or call a doctor. It also means you will be without staff for long periods so it is up to the residents to create their own entertainment, disability living allowance comes in very useful here.

Sheltered accommodation is a sort of 'half way house' between asylum and 'the real world' although generally not in my experience in an inner city or sink estate. It is a place for life so that you have some security, but they also encourage and provide help for you to move on. By having more independence than in hospital or an old style asylum, it is a useful stepping-stone to get back to independent living and leading ones own life. Unfortunately, not all residents will achieve this.

Living in sheltered accommodation has both social and private elements. This is of vital significance. If you feel unwell you can retire to your room or alternatively, if you need company, there will almost certainly be someone else who understands your illness or has had similar experiences to talk to. Staff will help you getting out and about and every year they accompany residents on holiday. A change of scenery is catered for thus giving you confidence that if a crisis occurs, the person will not be stranded miles away from help.

Thus such a job also requires that the staff can 'keep their heads' in a crisis, also a caring approach is needed and perhaps that the staff are not just 'doing it for the money'. They must know the right things to say in order to calm people down and prevent them from self-harm etc. However being able to listen as well as talk is just as important since, half the time, if you just listen to a person and give them 'someone to talk to' they will dissuade themselves from such actions. Furthermore, the project workers must be able to assess a situation and call a doctor if needed.

Staff must also be able to manage the inevitable conflicts that group living creates. There have been such problems ever since human beings first lived in societies. Indeed some people think there is no such thing as society. People are likely to get on each other's nerves and argue. On the other hand, such micro scale group living provides a supportive and friendly 'family' atmosphere. Living in such close confines despite the inherent problems this creates means you will get to know the other people very well indeed. Some people however think familiarity breeds contempt.

The key is the personality of the staff. Just

because some one has a degree in psychology does not make them the right person for the job. Such a person must have 'the knack' of being present in the background, to be there if needed, yet without being too intrusive and invasive of one's own privacy. This could be defined as 'people skills', but I think the best prerequisite experience is having also lived in a communal context (such as a hall of residence) for some time. Ultimately, the staff must become part of the family.

A correct choice of building is also important as there must be enough room for one's own personal space as well as a collective area in which to socialise. Ideally this would be something like a former old person's home but is more often a shared house. The advantage of the former over the latter is that there is more space both collectively and individually. It has been a government policy to encourage greater autonomy in such building design, by providing each room with a separate kitchen and bathroom. However such buildings can also create problems.

If a building, for example a former old people's home becomes inhabited by individuals who are obviously not old people, the neighbourhood will notice. This will be all the more obvious if cars are coming and going all day full of project workers, social workers and community psychiatric nurses etc. People will start wondering what is going on and sooner or later will find out that it is a mental health project with all the stigma that entails. Thus while such a context may be ideal in some ways, it can be problematic in others, although this might also be true of any such sheltered dwelling. On the whole, such contexts are in my experience very good places for the mentally ill and I would recommend it to everyone.

Life in an asylum.

Once upon a time, if you were admitted to a psychiatric hospital or 'asylum' (as it was generally referred to in the past) you would have stood some chance of becoming a long-stay patient. Life as a long-stay patient was however, very different to just being in hospital in a short-stay ward and I was lucky enough to get to see such a place first hand during a stay of more than a year. Indeed they the doctors were, at one point, also going to make me such a patient.

The criteria for being admitted as a long-stay patient are what are called 'enduring mental health problems' which are sometimes also called 'challenging needs.' This can cover a wide variety of reasons and difficulties but are used as a last resort. In my case, I had a tendency to wander around the countryside at night, to keep taking overdoses and (perhaps most serious of all) to forget to take my tablets. There were however also a couple of other young long-stay patients already at Winterton when I got there, so my case is not unique.

Despite having an image of the 'loony bin' and 'funny farm', life in Winterton was so good that some people did not want to leave. Hospitals can be wonderful places if the staff take the time to converse with and get to know the patients. Alternatively, if they do not adopt the hands on approach and prefer to stand back and observe, a stay in hospital can be very much the reverse. It seems that the location of the hospital has as much to do with this as the personality of the staff and can indeed be of central importance.

Winterton was a self-enclosed set of buildings on the edge of a small village and was even surrounded by a wall. Looking at these arrangements it seemed very reminiscent of a university campus! Most people however likened it to being a small village which, being from a remote small village myself; I also have to agree with. The parallel is the sense of community such a place generates by virtue of it's remoteness and self enclosure. Indeed people choose to go to this type of university or to live in the countryside often for these reasons as a commuter.

It was thought important that there would be a meeting place for patients to gather off the ward. This was to be therapeutic but was also meant to provide a 'space' for patients to get away from doctors and nurses. These facilities were thus staffed by non-medical personnel who knew little about psychiatry or mental illness. At Darlington Memorial Hospital, which is where Winterton was transferred to when it closed, there were plans to build such a place from the old hospital social club. This is extremely important.

The image of hospital as a self enclosed little world was not altogether correct. There was a restaurant and coffee shop which was open to the general public. This used to be the staff canteen but was turned into a business enterprise to make money and people would drive to the hospital just to go there. This allowed a bit of diversity, giving the feel of a normal coffee shop not full of patients and nurses, it also meant you had a choice between hospital food and the restaurant. The latter was much better than the former!

Long stay patients receive very little money and at one time were not allowed a television. This created a need for free entertainment. The entertainment was therefore extremely well organised and thought out; there was a non alcoholic bar, a minibus for outings, a fitness room, a church, a disco area (sometimes with singers), a place for watching cinema with a large screen, a library, pool tables, a little clothes shop and large grounds with playing fields, art therapy, and walking etc.

Life in hospital however was not all socialising and entertainment. There was no alcohol allowed in the bar and you had to be back on the ward at nine o'clock at night. If you wanted to go out of hospital grounds, it was necessary to ask permission. Long-stay patients are also expected to do some work such as in the laundry or washing dirty dishes. It even had a farm – made up of plant nurseries and allotments for this purpose. One's allowance was only fifteen pounds per week, half of which you were encouraged to save in a bank.

In hospital you are free to form relationships with whoever you wish. I always remember a patient telling me 'I always score whenever I go into hospital!' This happened to me a couple of times so it must be true!? Amazingly some people were not only married at the on site church (which still remains) but were also born in Winterton. This is hardly surprising given the community 'family' feel of such places.

Such hospitals are also full of history; they often date from Victorian times and thus have characteristic Gothic architecture although I found this a bit creepy! The wards had big old doors with large keys that looked like they were from a medieval dungeon. Some asylums were also former isolation hospitals for Leprosy and are thus even older, whilst doctors once upon a time really did wear white coats! Each year there was a group photo of the staff showing the evolution of such uniforms, which look very strange today.

One remnant of psychiatric history did disturb me however. At Winterton there was an operating theatre where a visiting surgeon would perform 'leucotomies' perhaps better known by it's American name – 'lobotomy'. It must have been a fairly common practice at one time, but thankfully rarely used today. One of the long-stay patients had such a procedure done and ended up with brain damage, it meant being dependent on hospital forever.

To sum up, I do like being out in the community but if I ever had to go back to Winterton I would. I have also heard that in America they are starting to build such places up again. All the more reason perhaps to inform people about them!

Institutionalisation and Rehabilitation.

Institutionalisation occurs gradually, often without with the patient ever really noticing. If it is noticed, (combined with other problems and fears) I suspect this can be a very frightening experience. Otherwise we can become so dependent that the fear only hits you when the doctor says you are ready to be discharged. This occurs by becoming familiar with the surroundings and environment particularly through the formation of friendships with staff and patients.

Being in hospitals in such close confines, we get to know the other patients in respect of friendship. This has a two fold effect. We can derive hope when we see people recovering and being discharged. Alternatively, we see people coming in and out (what staff refer to as the revolving door) which could be a cause for pessimism about recovery or the possibility of a relapse. Most often perhaps, we are pulled in both directions. Sometimes doctors and nurses become ill because of such an environment.

It is also possible, it has been suggested to me, to be drawn into other people's problems. This is difficult because although we are naturally sympathetic, it could worsen our own problems. Often wards have some very quiet patients and theoretically this may be one reason why. Alternatively sometimes friendships and even relationships are made with other patients and I have been told that this helps outside the hospital when discharged.

Seeing other ill people can remind you of your own problems. One patient suggested to me that it is best to get out of hospital as soon as possible to avoid such feelings. It has been commented to me that "every town and city should have a Waddington Street.". This should be the first port of call when coming out of hospital. This is for rehabilitation services.

A patient also commented that "I was going through the throws of daily routine but had no quality of life until going to Waddington street". It would seem from this, simply being able to cope is not enough to be discharged so there must be some social arrangement and activity to go to once 'outside.'

Hospital has been described by a patient very well as a "false environment." This is because everything is done for you. Outside you have to take responsibility so the longer the stay the greater these problems become. How then does this proceed?

The best thing to say about it is that it should be a gradual process, starting with the need for somewhere to go off the ward to avoid institutionalisation. This could be a café, another social function room or anywhere not surrounded by the doctors and nurses on whom we have depended on for help. This should be part of the hospital and the Winterton hospital I was in, had a number of such places including a cafe where members of the public could also go. Many people did so and it felt like being in a coffee shop in a town centre.

The problem here is that such developments would be very expensive for hospitals to institute. Darlington, for example were at one point going to spend £100,000 on such a development! They now have a brand new hospital instead. At some point (and how this is to be judged I am not sure) it will be necessary to leave hospital hopefully (as we have noted above) to a day centre.

There is also a funding question mark about how many places should be available and how long they should be open, especially at weekends. My local day centre is not able to do so financially which means going from Friday night to Monday morning without support. Sheltered accommodation could be relevant here but at some point it might be necessary or inevitable for the patients to rely on their friends and family or other patients.

The key is to keep busy. Being accepted as a person within a group at day centres is a good stepping-stone for being able to be part of a group in a work environment. We shall look at the rehabilitation process in more detail in the next section.

I wish to raise the question; "is 'Care in the community' with group living and day centres merely just another form of institutionalisation?" Many people express that they have little quality of life without such places whilst some even say that they are a veritable "life line." Institutions are cosy, like academics who nationally live in ivory towers, however, are we just creating a new form of dependency albeit in the real world? If this is the case, then the policy of 'Care in the community' will have failed in one of its main objectives, i.e. to restore our dignity and self-esteem by getting us back on our feet.

My own feeling about this that a new institutionalisation is created without the patient even knowing. We come to rely on day centres in the same way as we used to rely on hospitals. If they were taken away, how would people cope? Often, it is only one per cent of schizophrenics actually want to work. It seems therefore that whilst they may be 'able to survive out there', few achieve full independence. The answer may be to look at the issue more closely and try to remove the barriers to education and employment to solve this problem (I have written elsewhere on this subject).

The revolving door of re-admission.

My longest acute stay was for more than a year and I have had a
dozen admissions within eight years. Curiously, it has been pretty much the same each time, people sat around not talking to each other and just watching the "damn" TV! (which drives me to boredom). In one hospital I
was in, there was a lot of staff/patient contact, the influence of the ward sister I think. That made all the difference - a family
atmosphere, I guess with the same people on the 'revolving door', all
became part of the group of familiar faces which created a similar
feeling. After having been through the tread mill of sheltered
workshops, sheltered accommodation and then back to hospital, it gets to be
like more of a hotel than a hospital!

Of course, there was the occasional manic or psychotic episode,
but the strangeness within the social group seems to lessen over time
- you just get use to it. That, with knowing what all the medications
do, plus side effects, plus watching how the staff deal with the
thankfully rare crisis, you seem to end up looking at it the same way the
nurses do. Its just behaviour which requires

support, meds restraint
or whatever. I think I have absorbed the view of
the nurses a little
too much, but I hope this is an ethos of care.

I have had a few more thoughts from my
experiences here. I believe the nurses are not
meant to get too involved with the patients, but
this is difficult when you are watching someone in
acute distress. Moreover, after a years stay in
hospital where the compliment of nurses were
more or less the same, it becomes very difficult
indeed to keep that professional distance. This is
also true of sheltered accommodation and day
centres. Put any group of people in a room for a
year, they will get to know each other very well
indeed, those excluded by society and having
problems in common, seem to become reliant on
each other as
well.

It is supposed to be a caring profession, I once
had a girlfriend who was a general nurse and she
seemed quite idealistic about her work, at least
while she was training. I am sure there are
examples to the contrary but they seem
infrequent. People who are just "doing it for the
money" are perhaps unlikely to survive long in a
stressful, low paid job like that. In the end, 'MIND'
operate a ward watch system so that the worst
cases come under scrutiny.

There is one problem that does spring to mind and

that is of short staffing. Having to keep an eye on twenty or thirty patients limits how much time they can spend with you individually as a person. Also, I think the emphasis is much more on getting the medication correct than having a chat and being sociable, but without this, life on a mental health ward really would be hell. I have always managed to have some decent conversation with staff and patients but I have been ill so long I know them all quite well by now. Somewhere to socialise off the ward provides a good change of scenery, I have heard it suggested "a change is as good as a rest".

I have also been in a locked ward that was classed as an "intensive therapy unit." It was small with only five beds, but the close confines really made for a friendly, even close, relationship with the staff. There were three staff to five patients, I wish all wards had this ratio.

I was only in there for a week and that was enough for me. I did not really seem to notice the passage of time because I was so ill. Still, when I was released, I could almost smell the sense of freedom.

Up until very recently, our hospital was very utilitarian in furniture and food. The latter becomes of great significance when you are in for a long stay. It is one of the few things you begin to look forward to. Really, hospitals can be very boring sometimes.

None of the therapeutic activities were compulsory, except washing up, which got to be a pain in the neck after a year!

I am glad to say now, the beds, food and activities have all been greatly improved in our local hospital. This was a long time in coming. Now they have just got the meds to sort out!!

Activity Therapy.

When I was first asked to attend a therapy workshop in my local area, I was not convinced that it would help. This was because I had a strong educational background and thought I knew what it would be like. What a surprise I got.

At first glance, I thought the workshop would be too simplistic and that I would get bored very quickly. Indeed I had to be almost pushed into going by my social worker and family. The image of it was that it would be akin to factory work; i.e. something very monotonous and repetitive.

My first 'trial' day neither confirmed or changed this image but once I got to know the people and began to chat and socialise, the time seemed to fly. So much for first impressions. After a short time, I ended up going four days a week.

That was not the only surprise I was in for. At Broadgate farm I was asked to try my hand at art. My first reaction again, was that I had no artistic ability whatsoever, that I never could do it at school and even that I did not have the requisite gene as having an artistic 'bent' runs mystically within families.

So much for school! After being shown the theory of the vanishing point I ended up drawing and painting all sorts. Admittedly I was better at drawing buildings than spherical or irregular shaped objects and was better at painting than sketching, but so what?, I had achieved the seeming impossible!

The only problem is that I think you can have too much of a good thing. I also have a short attention span. Some measure of diversity in terms of activity, people and place was needed for me. I think therefore, a variety of locations and groups small enough to be a community but enough in number to give some diversity would be ideal.

I guess the moral of this story is; give the activities a try no matter what you think of them and how difficult they appear. It is true what they say "you never know until you have tried" and "don't judge a book by its cover", you might surprise yourself.

Activity at Christmas.

Christmas stereotypically tends to be a more difficult time of the year for anyone with a mental illness. This is perhaps because we have in mind, an image that every one is having a good time except me. A graphic illustration of this was provided by a friend who remarked; "oh you have to wear a smile on your face for two weeks." A cognitive approach is best here I believe, since it seems necessary to emphasize the positive aspects of Christmas

The image that everyone is 'enjoying themselves except me' is often not the case. There are plenty of other people who feel the same way about it. But looking at the Television over the festive period can give this impression. This thought however does not often help, so here are some others.

I try to avoid negative thinking about Christmas too much. For example "its just for the kids nowadays", "its just an excuse for getting drunk and overeating" and "its too commercialised" etc. This sort of thinking can reinforce an already depressed mind. Instead, if possible, look at some of the positives. Some reflection on the good this time of year brings out in people and the sense of community it creates, could give us the opportunity to be a part of it.

As I have family this positive thinking will be a lot

easier. You get excited for the kids when they get the Christmas presents – this is as much in the anticipation as 'seeing their faces.' Thus the buying and shopping for them is also just as good. I always try to treat myself as well, this is just as important!

Thus I also think the crowds add to the atmosphere despite the fact that city centres are all so busy. There used to be a coffee shop in Durham called 'Olivers'. You could sit upstairs watching people walk up and down 'Silver Street' through the window with the Christmas lights on. This was better than watching the TV! Very therapeutic and provided an opportunity for reflection.

I guess the real trick is getting to feel a part of things. We are socialised into it as a child and the good feelings we remember never really wear off. It is because of this that we feel left out if we do not have family contact of our own - we feel the emotional contrast. I have no wife and kids of my own but still enjoy Christmas tremendously.

Part of feeling depressed around Christmas could be 'Seasonal Affective Disorder' as December 21st is the year's shortest day. There is a guided walk around Durham that takes place on Christmas day for fresh air and exercise, which is useful against depression. This is not only interesting in itself but is also a very social thing to do. I think this is a novel alternative thing to do and is much better than it sounds and although I have never done it myself, I used to work in a pub on Christmas day and found it very therapeutic.

Finally, Christmas is meant to be a spiritual occasion, but it is often thought that this side has been lost as Christmas is too commercial, thus something has also been lost from the whole experience. Once however, I went to Midnight mass even though I am not routinely religious. I always felt hymns were too formal, but I loved the carol service. The whole place had a therapeutic atmosphere created by the music. I left feeling ready for the big day. Do not think "oh that will never work for me" or "I have been before" since you never know until you try!

Nobody pretends to have anything like the answer to these problems, but this is what Christmas means for me.

Coping Strategies.

Having both schizophrenia and depression can result in a curious situation for having coping strategies. This can be summarised by what could be described as 'a paradoxical' or 'contradictory' needs. The push is; that having depression can result in the need to get out and about instead of 'moping around the house all day'. Alternatively, what can impede this is the schizophrenic need to stay away from other people about which they are generally paranoid. The consequence is that the sufferer generally is pulled in both directions.

We have then the need to do both, i.e. stay at home and be away from home. We need then to do something to take our minds off the problem when away from home. However, this will very often not be possible and could require the need for a quick journey back in the event of a crisis, perhaps to consult a doctor or take medication. One's own transport may be needed here but often the sufferer will not be able to concentrate enough to drive safely

Exercise, it is often said, is the key to combating depression but in the context of a schizophrenic illness this is subject to the same problems as above when getting out and about. Taking a personal stereo to distract one's attention from the voices whilst out could help, however they can still be intrusive despite of this. Alternatively walking along a route frequented by buses to allow a quick escape home could also help. Failing that, having a mobile phone to ring for a taxi may be needed.

One problem even with these strategies is that during a psychotic episode we may have to act normal in front of the taxi or bus driver. It may thus be necessary to ring a support worker or relative instead. Panic attacks are a possibility if you are stranded 'miles away' from help. Having a mobile phone that allows you to see who you are talking to in such situations could also be useful here as you feel a calming effect by being able to be reassured by someone the sufferer trusts.

When suffering from depression it is vital to 'have something to get up in the morning for'. This could be any number of things but it must be something interesting, enjoying or otherwise satisfying to you however popular it may be for other people. This is something only you can do for yourself – nobody knows you as well as yourself. We must perhaps be open to suggestions here. In contrast, sometimes the answer to a period of mental illness is simply to go back to bed and sleep through it.

It may also be necessary to use what psychologists call 'positive reinforcement' on oneself. Thus we must remind ourselves that we are worthwhile human beings with many admirable qualities etc. This is to combat both low mood and voices which may be critical, both of which can undermine one's self esteem. Many mental health patients will already know and be familiar with this as 'cognitive behavioural therapy'.

The essence of one psychological approach is to keep a record of what one finds pleasurable and what one has accomplished (which is termed 'mastery'). Recording such experiences may thus serve to remind us that we do find certain things enjoyable, even if we do not often realise we do. By having such a focus introduced to us in this way, it is hoped that it will achieve this result.

Quite often, we will get good days and bad days and thus it is up to us to make the most of the good ones so that we can get over the difficult ones. Indeed some of the effort here has to come from the patient and so doing the house work for example (once we get cleaned up in the morning), we feel the better for it. Being bored and doing nothing can also affect one's mood. Even getting up in the morning however can require encouragement from someone else.

In the end however having mental health problems can be so overwhelming that any coping strategy can be to no avail, but until we try we will never know.

Life at day centres.

Day centres are a vital part of the 'Care in the community' programme. In the first instance, this is obviously because of the atomistic and anonymous nature of contemporary society and the stigma of being mentally ill. All of these problems I believe can be overcome. Thus day centres start as a lifeline and end up as a stepping-stone. You are being led down this path so subtly that you will almost be unaware of the process I am about to describe.

Initially I expected it to be something like hospital because all that was going on with regard to the very ill people on the ward was that there was nothing much to do but watch the television. On the ward the nurses had to tend to everyone and so could not focus on you at the expense of everyone else. There also did not seem to be very much contact with the other patients, although I did meet some very nice people in hospital.

At first, I thought I might 'give it a go' simply because coming out of the house would be a 'change of scenery', but would also be beneficial in that 'a change was as good as a rest'. There was nothing to lose by giving it a try even though this meant meeting new people and unfamiliar places. In my case there was no desperation involved arising from the nature of the society, I was more attracted by the prospect of learning about computers there. However, I suspect making the initial contact has for a lot of people as much to do with 'pull' factors than with 'push.'

My first impression was how busy it was. This creates a very social and friendly atmosphere rather like a coffee shop or a pub. It is also immediately obvious that everyone is enjoying themselves, including the staff. Unlike hospital, the people were animated and active. There was also no television – hurrah! People were actually talking to each other quite naturally, indeed it was hard to believe they were ill at all. I do not like to use the word, but it was also 'normal.'

Being in hospital prepares you for the social side in that there are both shared day rooms and shared bedrooms. People are brought together from all walks of life but have the same label put upon them by society so I think there is a natural tendency to group together and help one another. Diversity is not only the spice of life but rather like going to university as it broadens one's horizons. The people are just as interesting as the activities and they might also might include people from backgrounds you might not normally encounter.

One example for me stands out above the rest. Every Thursday night a professor of social policy hosts a drop in at my local day centre. However having being a postgraduate student myself, I know how difficult it is getting access to academics who have many demands on their time. Indeed I think most university students would give their right arm to have such lone access to a professor every week.

Having a life long illness means you will often see the same faces year in year out. This is beneficial because you get to know such people very well indeed. There is also a steady stream of staff and patients to provide a constant supply of 'new faces.' In this respect you have the best of both worlds.

Once you get involved in the activities, getting on the bus and coming to the centre begins to feel like commuting into town to get to a job. Together with integrating socially in the ways described above, you end up with all the necessary people and occupational skills to get back to work.

A local further education college runs the courses. This is significant in that once you get used to the teachers and how interesting it all is, the next step is easy. By this I mean going to the college itself is going more in-depth without having to be restricted to doing it at my local day centre. From here, getting back to work is not a massive leap.

In the end, the stigma ends up disappearing in that you end up making many friends and progressing to a social life outside the centre. If you go shopping, you are bound to bump into someone you know from the centre. This ends up overcoming the feeling of being isolated from the society because of the stigma. After a while the thought that you are the object of stigma not only simply fades into the background, but disappears completely.

Passing the time.

Becoming schizophrenic can change your whole life. You may be forced to change your job, lose your home and go into a hospital full of strangers. The patient however retains much of his identity minus some or all of these elements. The problem then becomes; how do you pass the time without work or family responsibilities? If you do not hear voices all day long there are going to be long gaps during which you can become very bored. Activity can become very distracting for a while, but can it replace the life that you have left behind?

Having interests outside of work is common. But I have found that you need something more substantial to 'fill your day.' Thus although I like Cds, DVDs, the internet and computer games, I cannot sit around the house all day with a remote control! This might seem surprising as to have this opportunity; most people I know would say "I would give might right arm to live like that!" I suspect if my experience is typical, such people would be in for a bigger surprise.

Inactivity breeds boredom and this ultimately makes you lazy. Everything becomes an effort and nothing seems to be worth the effort. In short, living like this gets to the point that you feel 'stuck in a rut'. It can get very depressing if not checked early on. Social workers and the like are clued up on this and will suggest some kind of therapeutic activity.

You can literally go from being a workaholic to a couch potato. It is just that your mind is wanting to go back to your life before the illness and cannot accept that any change is worth the effort. I guess it is necessary to avoid having 'tunnel vision' about life and try and try to adapt. This is not easy and the longer it all goes on the harder it is to get out of the 'rut' you find yourself in.

The problem is that we have already been through all this work and training at school. This however was not my problem because I loved school and university and planned on becoming an academic. The idea of creative therapeutic activity to fill my spare time was in this respect a dream come true! Thus I have done four years of part time Information Technology and an 'A' Level in Sociology. But I am still bored.

The cure for this came in the form of socialising with other people. To do this I had to start from scratch. Academics live in an ivory tower and apart from some part time bar work, I had never been in another environment. Going to the local drop thus took a long time to get to know every one.

Now I cannot stand to be at home for more than half an hour without recourse to my local day centre. At the weekend it is closed and this again creates big problems for me. I cannot socialise and have turned once again to the remote control.

It is all the more difficult because there is an anti-climax from having a relatively busy week.

At these moments you begin to dwell on your problems and when these include having a mental illness the impact can be huge. You start looking back on your life and thinking "what a waste". My CPN even thought that I was high at one point (during the week) and low at another (the weekend). I have not ended up with a diagnosis of bipolar however. At day centres you are taught to be expressive and creative - this is addictive. So much so that it begins to become your whole life and you want that creative feeling all the time. But life is not like that and it is only for a lucky few whom their job is also their hobby. You have to try to let it support your new life in this way.

The problem can arise I believe in the way society socialises you. At school you are taught to compete, to strive for high grades and prepare for life in this way. But having a mental illness robs you of this future and it can be very difficult (I find) to let yourself relax and put it on hold. Something has to fill the gap.

I have currently decided to write this book on mental health and this is beginning to occupy my time. The more practice the better and longer it seems to get and I have written about 25000 words in six months! I will keep you posted how I get on.

Education and the mentally ill.

As we have argued, there is a path for the mentally ill from day centres to college and then hopefully back into work. There are however a number of barriers to progression along this path. These are a vital part of the policy of social inclusion and are thus worth enumerating with a view to seeing what can be done to overcome them.

Some educational practice involves group work within a classroom context. But this would bring someone with schizophrenia into close proximity with strangers who may be the object of paranoia. It may however be better for people with depression because teamwork is a good way to break the ice and make new friends. In the case of schizophrenia, going as a group from a day centre and all enrolling on the same course could overcome this problem.

This is how teaching at 'Waddington Street' works – people sign up for courses in groups. If they go to a FE college as a group, it may help to increase people's confidence including being in class and answering questions. They could even help each other with the homework. They will also be able to have the confidence to socialise with other people on the course who are not ill –maybe!

In the beginning, it may be difficult to get the

energy needed to undertake a course of study. Often when you have had a long illness you get stuck in a rut. However it was in my case the more energy I expended the more I seemed to have, the whole thing became a virtuous circle. I even started to feel the competitive spirit of exams, which helps you move along the route back into employment.

What is required therefore is a kick-start to get the whole process started, i.e. a mixture of carrots and sticks. This might include financial incentives or arranging easy transport. Perhaps even an assistant on hand to help with homework after hours. The best incentive however, is to give a taste of learning which can act as a promise of similar things to come. Learning can be fun.

One particular problem is the possibility of relapse of a mental illness during a course. Thus you might miss out on say five or six weeks. Waiting to start the course again next year may cause the person to lose interest so it is important to get them back into learning as quickly as possible. This may require a bit of forceful persuasion. It may also be necessary to have some one-to-one tuition to catch up.

Also of relevance is the course structure. I did an 'A' Level while I was ill. It was beneficial to me that the course tutor began slowly and then quickened the pace with an increasing workload near to the exams at the end of the course. If you have not worked for a while, this sort of approach can be very useful for getting over the problem of becoming rusty.

One thought uppermost in my mind is; "what if I have a panic attack and embarrass myself in front of a whole class?" It may be necessary to have a nurse on duty like at Finchale college to provide a psychological security factor in the event of an emergency. Other symptoms like a period of hearing voices could be handled in class by going to the toilet for a while (but really going to see a nurse) or even going home and catching up with the lesson later.

It may look to the teacher that you are struggling and perhaps you might be better off dropping the course until you feel better. I did the advanced ECDL course at 'New College' in Durham and found it difficult to concentrate with my illness. I had to write everything down, do homework and even put posters up about subjects I kept forgetting. Despite all the obvious hard work, I passed and really enjoyed the whole experience. So do not be too quick to judge when you see someone trying too hard or making too much effort.

For me certain activities were more appropriate than others. Writing complex articles just to practice English skills might be too difficult, it may be better to teach this simply by pupils keeping a diary. I think creative crafts are a good contender too because doing art or pottery gives you a tangible physical product at the end of the day, but why I get this feeling about it I do not know. You hear a lot about computers these days, some students therefore may find IT interesting (they can also check your spelling which is an educational gremlin for many people). All these courses are covered at Waddington Street.

It is even a significant challenge becoming familiarised with the college building so people with a mental illness may need to have a guided tour. Especially important, is introducing the appointment and counselling service (where you can talk over problems). If you have never been in a class since school it might be worth just sitting in one during a lesson just to get the feel for it again.

It will need to be explained to the mentally ill person new to studying in this way, that subjects are full of technical words and references. The jargon can put people off so I feel some explanation that despite these academic features of social science subjects, its all just common sense and there is no need to be in awe of any of this. People will often have lots of life experience that they can draw upon which is of relevance to arts, humanities and social science. This should help from the point of view of building confidence.

One final point is that anti-psychotic medication makes you sleepy and this requires careful timing regarding getting up in the morning to go to class and doing homework in the evening etc. The drug I am on is Clozapine and, like clockwork, I sleep twelve hours every night. If the pupil looks tired in class it not because the are bored or lost its just the side effect of medication

Support suggestions.

One obvious support suggestion is a message board on the college website is accessible only to students who have a mental health problem. Such a service is available on a Channel 4 website, it should serve as a way for students to share their experiences and talk about their own barriers to education.

Another idea is that there could be a special rest room for pupils who are ill and feel they need somewhere to relax, be entertained or talk over their problems with people with the same difficulties. This, like mental health day centres in towns, should foster a supportive group identity and manufacture supportive friendships within the college.

In a crisis situation, it may be best to have a CPN on hand in the rest room to provide someone to talk to. The problem there is going to be that you can only be referred to hospital by your local G.P. This is a huge potential barrier for very ill students who may feel they are going out of area to go to college. In such situations, the immediate thought in the students mind may be getting into hospital as quickly as possible.

Sometimes it may not be possible for a student to get to college through feeling too paranoid. They may still want to learn however. Some e-learning with one-on-one teacher video conferencing could prevent the student falling behind on such days.

There will still have to be some guidelines about how long a student can go on missing a course before one-on-one supervision will become ineffective in allowing the student to catch up. If the student does get to the end of the course but fails the exams, there will be a need to intervene to support the results as they might be taken rather badly. Revision meanwhile, is particularly stressful and thus might require extra educational and therapeutic support as well.

Introduction to the often unfamiliar learning environment is an important issue. It may be necessary to be shown around by a student who has mental health problems and has successfully achieved a full time course at the same institution. This will give the patient the opportunity to ask questions the access committee may not have thought of. Seeing is believing and this should inspire confidence. An alternative prospectus for students with mental health problems recording such instances may also be required.

Fear and confidence are the two greatest barriers to learning. A pre-course induction programme may be necessary comprising teaching social skills, cognitive barriers to getting into education (e.g. removing preconceived ideas such as "it will be too hard"). Such a pre term programme could also include getting the feel of sitting in a class with other students, talking to the course tutors and giving a sample lesson. This will be a learning experience for the staff as well.

It could just be like at Waddington Street, i.e. some courses should be run just for the mentally ill. Such problems are so common it might be a viable proposition in terms of class size. Mentally handicapped people work in this way at new college. Again this would remove socialising barriers to learning.

College as an institution, is itself a supportive environment. All the time having a mental illness involves a series of institutions, i.e. (in order) hospital to sheltered accommodation to day centres to New College itself. Along this path we are constantly having to adapt though we may still have psychological barriers about "going somewhere new" or "a place full of strangers". Some reflection should help overcome these cognitive difficulties and once they "get used to it" it will become a source of psychological security.

Some education of the staff might reassure the student they are in a safe environment and indeed schizophrenia will be mentioned on courses in sociology and psychology. It may be also better to go to college on an evening course, where there are more mature students who may have themselves more knowledge about mental health (though I am not sure what the research on this is). The evening is a good time for one-on-one learning to catch up on periods which have been missed.

Barriers to educating the mentally ill tend to vary from individual to individual. What is not needed is some universal approach, but a range of options and considerations dependent on the personality and experiences of each student.

The most obvious barriers arise from people's memories of school. If these are positive (and that is generally the case) prior to a mental illness then motivation, confidence and enthusiasm for education are likely to be high, but if their experience was negative it may be necessary to look at experiences of work instead and direct the student towards a more vocational course.

As we have said, reactions to school are crucial. This is because it is "the time before the illness." What you get is a series of attitudes and assessments of the school experience. These range from trauma to monotony to instrumentality (to get a job). People will say "I loved school except for physical education", "I wish I paid more attention at school", "I hated school but I did like Chemistry", "I used to be good at school but wish I could have took it further." Changing the way the student thinks about education cognitively seems very important and might have to involve an education psychologist.

In my case I had a break down followed by depression whilst still at university. Even at my lowest point, I was able to work academically. I just tried to ignore my problems and eventually they went away. Keeping my work up thus provided a focus away from what was happening to me and gave me a valuable sense of normality. This was better for my esteem. I have even been in hospital and enrolled on a basic computer course. A course in exercise at college was good for my depression and should also be provided by the college.

What concerned me most however, was the need to keep up appearances. I was always wondering whether anyone could tell. I was stigmatised by the thought of going to the counselling service and even though I needed help, I thought I had to deal with my problems myself. The biggest barrier to education here is to educate about the stigma so that the student seeks out help. Mental health within college should have a high profile. Perhaps putting posters with song lyrics from well-known pop songs will help to do this best!

In the case of my own schizophrenia, I felt the whole society was against me. Going to college however, was something I was used to and was not just good therapy but helped me reintegrate with society by providing a normal social context and activity. It helped my hang on to my sanity even when I was at my most ill. Thus, I believe it is possible for some to study even during a crisis.

In the end it is up to the student.

Family and Friends.

An acquaintance pointed out to me that when she developed her mental illness, she was afraid to tell her friends and family because of the social stigma. She also noted that whilst some people may think like this, society did provide the NHS, education and social services. However, in one recent 'Mind' survey, 33% of respondents felt that family and friends reacted differently to them because of the media image of madness. Thus, I feel it is necessary to look at the issue in more detail.

Often, people with a mental illness dare not tell their friends and family about their problems. This has a long history. In the past, if there was ever a 'history of insanity' in the family, it was never talked about. Being cut off from one's family whilst ill can be very detrimental to the need for therapy and could also cause depression (in addition to other problems). This is all the more serious when such an illness carries a stigma and thus severs the link with society as well.

From a theoretical point of view, there are different opinions. Some people think there is no such thing as society, only individuals and families. This would tend to magnify the therapeutic importance of the family. Another view is that of R.D. Laing who thought that the family could cause schizophrenia. Another view of what are called the 'sociological functionalists' think that the family is like getting into a warm bath which functions as a support for coping with life's problems. These views are in need of some illustration.

Family life (as we all know) is not often all it should be even taking into account the problems raised for it by its members having a mental illness. Edward Leach, also a sociologist, described the family as an 'overloaded circuit' in which "huddled together in their loneliness, the parents fight and the children rebel." Thus the figures for domestic violence are 25% and the divorce rate is 40% of all marriages (with an extra 20% just staying together for the sake of the kids). All this limits the potential therapeutic content of family relation and marriage.

Often geographical distance is a factor in considering family contact. In technical terms this is described as being the difference between a 'nuclear' and an 'extended' family, i.e. the former composed of mother, father and children the latter made up of grand parents, aunts and uncles. There is some disagreement among sociologists about what the trends are, but all agree both types of family form exist. Despite geographical distances being involved and other difficulties in getting to see one's relatives because of work etc, there remains, sociologist argue, the ever increasing importance of progress in communications and travelling which makes some of the distances involved less of a factor. However, nothing can substitute for being in the same physical space.

It may be thought that family life itself is under threat as there has been an increase in people having a series partners and children but not getting married. This has been defined as 'creative singlehood' and 'serial monogamy.' There is thus less family contact in the sense that people can rely on their partners for support when developing a mental illness. The picture in general is not so bleak however: 80% of divorced couples remarry within a short period of time. Family life is still the norm despite these changes although they are significant enough to warrant a new label. Robert Chester calls it "the neo-conventional family."

The possible effects of 'family life' on the mentally ill thus seem to form a spectrum between two very different extremes that I call 'care' and 'cruelty.' The worst example of 'cruelty' I know of is that of a young lady who was sexually abused by her father and developed schizophrenia (although not necessarily as a result of this). She began hearing voices and these voices were those of her family members, including her father. Here therefore family relations have been very damaging in terms of mental health.

At the other extreme is that of T.L.C. (tender loving care). It is perhaps the hardest thing in the world to watch their own child go through all the terror and suffering associated with having a mental illness. Often in such times friends will 'show their true colour' although the other possibility is that our 'fair weather friends' will desert us and we will see 'who our true friends are'. I am not sure that this last point is altogether true even if our friends do desert us.

This is again because of the pervasive nature of the social stigma surrounding mental health problems. This creates all kinds of problems for ones friends and family, including reactions ranging from fear and hostility to ridicule and shame. If these attitudes are so deeply rooted in our culture then I do not believe one's friends and relatives are to blame for reacting the way they do. This calls for a massive publicity drive in the media to reduce the stigma targeted especially at the family.

R.D. Laing for his part, thought that arguing parents were responsible for causing schizophrenia in children. He describes the situation of the child as "being batted like a ping pong ball" between arguing parents. This forces the child to escape into a fantasy realm, at which point schizophrenia develops. The predominant theory nowadays is a medical one and it is something which genetic research is giving added weight to. Nevertheless, Laing is still influential today in what is called 'The anti-psychiatry movement'.

In spite of all this theory and science, it seems to me, that the bond of family life is one of the strongest emotional forces that human beings can experience. Having support from one's family is thus absolutely critical. In this respect, it can perhaps also lead us to question things like paranoia and depression. Alternatively, if we lack such a situation or background then we are very often lost, isolated and alone and as a consequence our mental health problems will be much worse.

The effects of mental illness on families.

The initial development of a mental illness can be particularly terrifying given that very little is known about it by the population at large. What people are more aware of is the stigma. Often people will be dissuaded from seeking help for this reason. It will become obvious however that the sufferer will be behaving unusually and perhaps will also be evasive about why. Here then hopefully, the family must step in and call a doctor. This is the beginning of a series of possible emotions, reactions and events that affect both the sufferer and the family.

To see loved ones suffering a mental illness is probably one of the hardest things to endure. Parents naturally worry about their children but having a mental illness is certainly having something to worry about. Perhaps the central concern is that the sufferer will commit suicide. As a result, relatives inevitably begin to probe and question the situation in which they find themselves, this leads to a series of steps by which they find out about it.

It will appear to the parent that the mentally ill person does not understand what is going on around them. There is thus a gap of communication, which no amount of explanation and persuasion can bridge. The sufferer therefore appears isolated and helpless; this can be a particularly distressing thought for all involved.

Experiencing a mental illness is also something that is hard to understand and explain from the subjective point of view of the sufferer. This leaves a gap, which can perhaps have both a positive and negative effect on relatives, positive if the symptoms are worse than their outward signs and negative if vice versa. This gap however is often a source of some worry in itself regarding the severity of the condition.

It is also hard sometimes for the parent to be able to offer emotional support because the delusions and paranoia can cut one off (even from one's own kin) in another way, e.g. if they form the focus of some of the psychotic symptoms. The thought that the person is again suffering alone is particularly distressing and is perhaps a unique possibility to this kind of illness.

Often if a section is needed, a parent's consent is required. This can cause some tension. It may be that the person will try to dissuade the parent from doing this, especially if the section too is a source of paranoia. In such cases the police will be called and the ensuing struggle will be all the more distressing for all concerned.

Another factor often uppermost in the mind of the parent is the likelihood of a cure. The professionalism of the doctors and of the other medical staff here is high and is likely to impress. Unfortunately, the statistics for the recovery rate are not so quite impressive and eventually it will all too often become obvious that the illness is likely to be ongoing, which requires the support of the family.

The onset of all this can also come as a shock. Everyone hears of cases of mental illness in the media but the thought is always that 'it will never happen to me'. The effect is like that of a sudden awakening with a subsequent gradual process of coming to understand and accept what is happening. Fortunately here there is a wealth of information available in books and on the internet.

Life is full of ups and down and if the onset of a relative's psychiatric illness occurs when things are difficult or even during a time of crisis, then it can be all the more distressing. I suppose the extreme example is that it may trigger such an illness in the sufferer's own relatives. Under such circumstances, this is most likely to be a slight or perhaps temporary case of depression but could even be a psychotic reaction. Stress can also be the cause of such a reaction.

Nevertheless there is a vast support network of organisations and groups. The most well known is 'Mind' - offering advice, information and other help for relatives of sufferers of mental health problems. These will aid with the processes and difficulties of understanding the illness from the experience of health professionals but also from the experiences of sufferers, including those who have recovered. Seeing such cases 'in the flesh' can be invaluable and will help overcome the problems in understanding outlined above.

It also provides an opportunity for relatives to share the weighty burden as well as providing support for those caring for someone with a mental illness. It will also be a context in which the stigma of the illness will quickly be dispelled and an appreciation of how common and 'normal' such problems are, despite public image of the condition. Ultimately such groups will provide a channel of feedback to the medical establishment thus also making relatives feel they have some influence in the treatment sufferers receive.

What results from this process ultimately, is the hope that there will be some medical breakthrough that will cure the sufferer or at least prevent him or her from self-harm or suicide. Sadly this cannot be guaranteed. An important point however, is that even the most 'particularly severe' cases can be cured outright, so that from a parent's perspective this group contact and the line of thought involved can be a very positive outcome indeed.

Milton Keynes UK
Ingram Content Group UK Ltd.
UKHW030719300824
447605UK00001B/7

9 781847 470973